'This book draws together a broad range of chapters and authors about the less explored, because considered obvious, concept of space in dramatherapy. Especially innovative areas for me were scenography and ritual space, in addition to the useful chapters on educational and play spaces. This book opens up a dialogue about the many spaces among, between and with which we work as dramatherapists. Trainees, practitioners and researchers can usefully develop their own perspectives from this invaluable volume'.

**Ditty Dokter, PhD,** *past course leader MA dramatherapy,*
*Roehampton and Anglia Ruskin Universities*

W0234979

# Space, Place and Dramatherapy

*Space, Place and Dramatherapy: International Perspectives* provides radical, critical and practical insights into the relevance and significance of space and place in dramatherapy practice. Bringing together an international breadth of contributors, the chapters of this book reveal extensive reflections on the many spaces in which dramatherapists and their clients work and offer research implications for those wishing to critically examine their own symbolic or structural spaces in dramatherapy practice.

Chapters consider space and place from many angles: ritual and symbolic spaces; transitional and play spaces; educational and interpersonal spaces; and scenographic and architectural spaces. The book examines the impact of space on human (and more-than-human) relationships, dramatherapy practice and processes and mental health, offering new avenues of research and critical enquiry.

This volume is the first of its kind to rigorously elucidate the importance of space within the field of dramatherapy and is essential reading for academics, scholars and postgraduate students of dramatherapy, as well as practicing dramatherapists and professionals within the wider domains of arts and health.

**Eliza Sweeney** is a lecturer in art therapy at the University of Caen, France, and the University of Melbourne, Australia, in art therapy. She is a dramatherapist, scenographer, artist and PhD researcher at the University of Northumbria.

# Routledge Research in Creative Arts and Expressive Therapies

This series provides a forum to discuss the latest research, debates and practice in creative arts and expressive therapies; including arts therapy, dance therapy, dramatherapy and music therapy.

**Intercultural Music Therapy Consultation Research**
Shared Humanity in Collaborative Theory and Practice
*Lisa Margetts*

**Reflections on Authentic Movement**
Theory, Practice and Arts-Led Research
*Eila Goldhahn*

**Space, Place and Dramatherapy**
International Perspectives
*Edited by Eliza Sweeney*

# Space, Place and Dramatherapy
International Perspectives

**Edited by Eliza Sweeney**

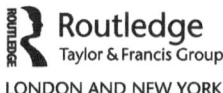
Routledge
Taylor & Francis Group

LONDON AND NEW YORK

First published 2024
by Routledge
4 Park Square, Milton Park, Abingdon, Oxon OX14 4RN

and by Routledge
605 Third Avenue, New York, NY 10158

*Routledge is an imprint of the Taylor & Francis Group, an informa business*

*British Library Cataloguing-in-Publication Data*
A catalogue record for this book is available from the British Library

ISBN: 978-1-032-16939-2 (hbk)
ISBN: 978-1-032-17234-7 (pbk)
ISBN: 978-1-003-25239-9 (ebk)

DOI: 10.4324/9781003252399

Typeset in Galliard
by MPS Limited, Dehradun

In 2016, as a young and enthusiastic dramatherapy Masters' student, I assisted at the second European Dramatherapy Federation conference in Romania where I presented my first conference paper on space and place in dramatherapy.

I was sure I had been able to make my 'brilliant' point come across but afterwards I found myself in a lively discussion with Scottish, David Keir Wright. While I was arguing that the subject matter of space and place in dramatherapy required deeper thought and research, David claimed it was an 'obvious' fact. Loosely referring to Arthur Conan Doyle, I replied vigorously that 'there is nothing more deceptive than an obvious fact' and by this reminding David and myself that research is nothing if not bringing to light the intricacies and hidden crucial effects of seemingly mundane or obvious phenomena.

I pause here to acknowledge my deep respect for David who is no longer with us. My banter with him only gave me confidence and strengthened belief to embark on this book project. I felt him challenging me at that time was proof of an elder respecting me and taking my wholehearted passion for the subject matter seriously.

It is with great sadness for me that David will not be reading this book or would have contributed with a chapter that maybe he would have titled 'The obviousness of space in drama therapy', but I hope he is with us in spirit and I am forever grateful to him.

This book is dedicated to David.

# Contents

*List of Figures*                                                      *xi*
*List of Tables*                                                      *xii*
*About the Contributors*                                            *xiii*
*Foreword*                                                           *xvi*
*Preface*                                                             *xx*
*Acknowledgements*                                                *xxiii*

Prelude: The Obviousness of Space of Anything But                      1
ELIZA SWEENEY

**PART 1**
**The Built Environment and Scenography in**
**Dramatherapy**                                                      15

1 Teachings from Echo                                                 17
ELLEN FOYN BRUUN

2 How Hut-Making in Dramatherapy Created a
Therapeutic Play Space                                               29
ANGIE RICHARDSON

3 Space Plays a Leading Role: The Therapeutic Power of
the Built Environment and Co-Design in Dramatherapy                  42
ELIZA SWEENEY

4 Neutral Mask and Embodied Dreamwork, Spaces of
Containment                                                          60
MAYRA STERGIOU

**PART 2**
**Education and Play Space in Dramatherapy**                     73

  5  Learning and Therapeutic Spaces in Dramatherapy and
     Education                                                     75
     CLIVE HOLMWOOD

  6  Connecting Spaces: Playing to Relate                          91
     SARAH MANN SHAW

  7  Essential Factors Both Practical and Imaginal for
     Defining the Dramatherapy Play Space in Special
     Education                                                    104
     AMANDA MUSICKA-WILLIAMS

**PART 3**
**Ritual, Intersubjective and Spiritual Space**                 121

  8  The Fullness of Emptiness: The Significance of Space
     and the Usefulness of the Concepts of *Shunya* (The
     Void/Empty Space), *Akasha* or *Vyoman* (Open
     Vastness), *Kha* (The Enclosed Space) in Hinduism and
     Buddhism for Dramatherapy Practice                          123
     BRUCE HOWARD BAYLEY

  9  'Clear the Space. Claim the Space. Sanctify the Space':
     Intersubjectivity and Spirituality in Dramatherapy
     According to Roger Grainger                                 137
     SALVO PITRUZZELLA

10  Liminality and Ritual in Dramatherapy – The
     Intersubjective Space                                       149
     JOANNA JAANISTE

11  Preparing the Ritual Space: The Transition from
     Everyday Reality to Dramatic Reality                        162
     DREW BIRD

     Postlude: Future Spaces of Dramatherapy                     176
     ELIZA SWEENEY

     *Index*                                                      183

# Figures

5.1  A description of liminal dramatic and therapeutic space          79
5.2  Amorphas and elastic single-cell dramatherapy space             80
8.1  Meditation hall, Karla temple cave, Maharashtra, India          132

# Tables

3.1  The Object-to-Client Observation Table                                          52
5.1  Distance Model of Dramatherapy                                                  84
7.1  Contrasting Examples of the Ways in Which the Space is Set Up
     to Meet Differing Needs of Participants in Special Education          111

# Contributors

**Bruce Howard Bayley,** England, is an Indian-born Anglo-Indian Dramatherapist, based in Central London who has been working widely and specifically with survivors of addictions, sexuality, self-harm, sexual, physical and spiritual abuse and psychological trauma. He has presented papers and workshops (including his own Tribhuvan Threefold Psycho-spiritual Dramatherapy) in the United Kingdom, Nürtingen, Milan, Warsaw, Beijing, Mumbai, Chennai and Pune. He has been associated with a number of UK universities as a trainer, supervisor and external examiner with a special interest in multicultural clinical practice and working with marginalized populations.

**Drew Bird,** U.K. has been a Dramatherapist for twenty years. He was senior lecturer on the MA in Dramatherapy at the University of Derby for fifteen years. He is currently associate professor and senior lecturer at the University of Melbourne, Australia where he teaches on the MA in Drama therapy. He was editor of the Dramatherapy Journal from September 2020 to March 2023. He is currently co-editing a book on dramatherapy and spirituality. He is the author of 15 publications and editorials. Recent research interests and publications have focussed on heuristic inquiry, arts-based research and a/ r/ tography. He presents at conferences internationally. His background is in working with children and young people who have experienced trauma and adult mental health. He is also in private practice.

**Ellen Foyn Bruun,** Norway, is a dramatherapist trained in the Sesame Approach to drama and movement therapy, University of London. She is a Professor of Drama and Theatre at the Norwegian University of Science and Technology, NTNU Trondheim. Over the last decade she has pioneered dramatherapy in Norway and the Nordic countries through teaching, research and intersectional networking of Arts and Health. Her professional background is stage directing, playwriting/dramaturgy and drama teaching. Her research and teaching practice seeks to explore and develop practice that contributes to personal and artistic insight and learning for promoting health and wellbeing. She is an Associate teacher of Fitzmaurice Voicework® and one of research interests explores the integration of voicework in dramatherapy and performance on and off the theatre stage. She is an active contributor to international and European dramatherapy communities and has published several articles, written plays and contributed to books on dramatherapy, voicework and theatre practice.

**Clive Holmwood,** United Kingdom, is a Dramatherapist with 25 years of experience and an Associate Professor in the Discipline of Therapeutic Arts, University of Derby. He lectures and researches in Dramatherapy and Creative Arts Health and well-being with an interest in the development of drama education, dramatherapy and play. His PhD from the University of Warwick was published by Routledge in 2014 as '*Drama Education and Dramatherapy*'. He co-edited *Learning as a Creative and Developmental Process in Higher Education*, Routledge and co-edited a trilogy of Routledge International Handbook's, *Dramatherapy* (2016) *Play, Therapeutic Play and Play Therapy* (2020) and Therapeutic Stories and Storytelling (2022). He is a Neuro-Dramatic Play Practitioner and Trainer and runs a private dramatherapy practice – Creative Solutions Therapy Ltd.

**Joanna Jaaniste,** Australia, is an Australian dramatherapist with 29 years of experience. An Adjunct Fellow of Western Sydney University, she has worked for 22 years with adults in the mental health system. A trauma-informed therapist, she has experience with people who have substance abuse and adolescents at risk. She has a small private practice working with clients and supervisees. Her main research is in dementia, and she has published widely including writing a book on this topic, also lecturing and presenting her work in Europe, the United States of America and South Africa. She has until recently been a board member of the World Alliance of Dramatherapy.

**Sarah Mann Shaw,** United Kingdom, is a dramatherapist and psychotherapist working in private practice in the UK. She has extensive experience of working with children and adolescents alongside statutory and private agencies. She works with the impact of disrupted attachments and trauma using dramatherapy. She has two articles published in the Dramatherapy Journal, 'Metaphor, Symbol and the Healing Process in Dramatherapy' (1996), and 'The Drama of Shame' co-written with Di Gammage (November 2011). She has a chapter in Routledge International Handbook of Dramatherapy (2016) and is contributing a chapter to Dramatherapy and Neuroscience (2021).

**Amanda Musicka-Williams,** Australia, is trained as a drama and movement therapist at the Central School of Speech and Drama in London. She has practiced dramatherapy in Australia for 18 years, working with a diverse range of client groups including students in mainstream and special education, adults in mental health care settings, prison systems and homeless support services. She recently completed doctoral research exploring relationships and interpersonal learning through group dramatherapy with adolescents in special education.

**Salvo Pitruzzella,** Italy, is a pioneer of dramatherapy in his country, founder of the first training in dramatherapy at the 'Centro ArtiTerapie', Lecco, Italy. He is a Retired Professor of Arts Education at the Fine Arts Academy of Palermo, Italy. He is Honorary Member of the EFD (European Federation of Dramatherapy); Member of Executive Board of the SPID (Società Professionale Italiana di Drammaterapia); International Member of the BADTh (British Association of Dramatherapists), and member of the Editorial Advisory Board of the Dramatherapy Journal. He has widely published on dramatherapy, educational theatre and creativity theories, including Drama, Creativity and Intersubjectivity, Routledge 2016.

**Angie Richardson,** New Zealand, is a clinically registered Creative Arts therapist and registered primary school teacher in Aotearoa, New Zealand. She has been a Lecturer in the Master of Creative Arts Therapy programme at Whitecliffe. She has a private practice working with children, teens and adults and contracts her services to schools and organizations. Her passion for dramatherapy stems from having run a drama school for children, many years of free-form improvization training and play sessions with profound personal healing from this modality. She believes in the alchemy and magic of the expressive arts to empower people to find their soul medicine.

**Mayra Stergious,** Greece, is a Theatre Director, Performer, Scenographer and Dramatherapist. She trained in Lecoq method at the London International School of Performing Arts (LISPA) and in Dramatherapy at University of Derby (2012). In 2012, she co-founded Vertebra Theatre, an ensemble focusing on creating contemporary Physical and Visual Theatre where she is the Artistic Director since. She has been teaching workshops on Devised Physical Theatre, Neutral Mask and Puppetry internationally. She is currently an Associate Lecturer at MSc Creative Computing at the University of the Arts (London) and undertaking a PhD at Guildhall School of Music & Drama researching Visual Theatre and Trauma.

**Editor, Eliza Sweeney,** France-Australia, holds an MA in Dramatherapy from the University Paris Descartes, and an Advanced Diploma of Neuro-Dramatic-Play. She is currently the recipient of a full PhD scholarship (RDF) from the University of Northumbria in Architecture. She explores therapeutic design within the global environmental crisis. She was the French representative in the European Federation of Dramatherapy for two years. She is a visiting lecturer on the MA in Creative Arts Therapies at the University of Melbourne, Australia, and on the MA in Psychology at the University of Caen, France. Her most recent publications are 'A Space of Their Own: A case-study advocating appropriation of the domestic interior for well-being' (2022) and 'Solastalgia, sense and therapeutic ecoscenography' (2022). This is her first edited book.

# Foreword

It gives me great pleasure to welcome this new book on Dramatherapy Space: *Space and Place and Dramatherapy: International Perspectives* by Eliza Sweeney. It is refreshing to find new ideas within a profession that is often preoccupied with roles and characters, scenes and stories.

The poem 'Down the glimmering staircase' by Siegfried Sassoon takes us into a world of childhood space – both for the child as well as the adult remembering early times past. The poet writes 'childhood creeps on tiptoe' and then creates poignant atmosphere by describing a staircase that glimmers and a clock that is pensive. He introduces the idea of escaping from the restrictive house into the freedom of the garden. But then it goes further, the train, 'night's last goods train going', takes the child, us and the child in us, into a land beyond the limitations of the orchard and the pond:

'Tells of earth untravelled and what lies beyond
Catching roach and gudgeon in the orchard pond'.

Sassoon takes us into special spaces in this poem, just like this important and unique book: *Space, Place and Dramatherapy: International Perspectives*. The book, edited by Eliza Sweeney, has 11 chapters by international specialists, who work in a variety of settings.

The text is divided into three definitive parts, dealing with contrasting spatial themes:

1 The built environment and scenography in dramatherapy
2 Education and play space in dramatherapy
3 Ritual, intersubjective and spiritual space

Each author describes the space in which they work together with their own beliefs and theory about therapeutic, educational and spiritual space. Very importantly, several authors address the theme of ritual and its important function in dramatherapy and spirituality. It was only in my own studies in becoming an anthropologist, that I fully understood the importance of ritual and its function in all spheres of our lives. Dispense with rituals and life for many becomes chaotic and disorganized, boundaries become dissolved and life transitions collapse.

In the first part, The Built Environment and Scenography in Dramatherapy, there are four chapters which look at several settings and age groups. In Chapter 1, Ellen Foyn Bruun writes about the space between dramatherapy and voice, and her understanding of space is 'experiential and emergent'. She not only refers to spatial metaphors but also 'material phenomena relating to being ourselves, others and the world'. Having trained in voice work with the Roy Hart Theatre, she suggests we communicate outwards in play and drama. She draws our attention to aural perception as contrasted with visual perception: echo as contrasted with Narcissus. She suggests that the visual is usually dominant in our thinking and reminds us that the 'space before language is sound'.

Angie Richardson's chapter describes her work with children through the Maori myth 'How Maui slowed the Sun'. The space is not therapeutic with other adults coming in and out, yet the children are immersed in hut-making (whare in Maori). She makes a fascinating observation 'I also noted how quickly shyness and hesitation can dissipate in the spirit of such conspiratorial play'. She is referring to the fact that the children were climbing on chairs and tables which was 'not allowed'!

Eliza Sweeney discusses the importance of the scenography of the dramatherapy room, emphasizing that it is more than decoration and function, 'We are "doing" space as much as space is doing things to us'. She gives several client vignettes, one, in particular, illustrates her main thrust of the importance of the space, when a client made use of a fabric curtain as a transitional object.

Mayra Stergiou writes about her work with adult prisoners within the prison institution. She makes use of the neutral mask and observed that through the wearing of a neutral face, the participants were able to get in contact with their inner space, their inner landscape. They were able to switch off self-censorship and what she terms their 'inhibitory selves'.

Part Two: Educational and Play Space in Dramatherapy

Clive Holmwood discusses the 'space within the space' and how clients we find challenging maybe finding the dramatherapy space a challenge! Often they experience their outside world as conforming and repetitive, is it possible for the dramatherapy space to reflect their needs and be more flexible? Holmwood draws upon Caldwell Cook and Slade to remind us that play is the core of dramatherapy: the space between the everyday and the dramatic, the empathy and the distancing; is it too close or too far? The space must be believable for therapy and education, for the drama and the learning. And it may change at a moment's notice!

Sarah Mann Shaw contributes a chapter with the title 'Connecting Spaces. Playing to Relate'. She discusses an example of Billie, a child who was removed at birth and placed with foster parents, who were 'relationally inconsistent'. She quotes Meares who talks about the 'poetry of making relationships'. She says the poetry of dramatherapy is in the playful encounter. She reminds us of Rogers's three core growth conditions: genuineness, unconditional positive regards, and accurate empathy.

Amanda Musicka-Williams writes on 'Essential Factors Both Practical and Imaginal for Defining the Dramatherapy Space in Special Education'. She suggests there are four types of space: psychological, physical, imaginal and intersubjective/relational. She emphasizes that the dramatherapy space must be safe and private. We are reminded that the crucial element of hide and seek is the being found! Our attention is also drawn to the importance of imitation, the learning that takes place through the copying of roles.

The third part of this book is Ritual, Intersubjective and Spiritual Space. Bruce. H. Bayley writes a very moving chapter entitled 'The Fullness of Emptiness. The Significance of Space and the Usefulness of the Concepts of Shunya, Akasha or Vyoman, Kha in Hinduism and Buddhism for Dramatherapy Practice'. He sees questions relating to identity that also connect to location.

- Who or what is to change?
- Where does the process take place?
- What relationship does the client/therapist have to the space? How does the client/therapist contribute to the process?
- May liminal space be considered useful or not in facilitating the therapy process?

With groups he observed anger and rage turning to something tender; the individual's anger – guilt and rage; from closed in attitude to serenity, from resentment to acceptance.

Salvo Pitruzzella's chapter is a touching tribute to the important work of Roger Grainger, who died tragically before his time: 'Clear the Space – Claim the Space, Intersubjectivity and Spirituality in Dramatherapy According to Roger Grainger'. Space is dramatic, therapeutic and sacred. 'Space is a ... vibrant and meaningful co-constructed microcosmos, created by human relationships and serving them, and endowed with a spiritual ego-transcending value'. Betweenness is the space that divides and connects, being with the other while not becoming then other. It is theatrically and philosophically founded.

This chapter connects beautifully with 'Liminality and Ritual in Dramatherapy – The Intersubjective Space' by Joanna Jaaniste. She considers how entry, exit, objects and props all play roles in the relational interpersonal space. The liminal experience is defined by ritual, warm-ups, action and reflection.

The final chapter by Drew Bird is 'Preparing the Ritual Space: The Transition from Everyday Reality to Dramatic Reality'. He discusses the preparation of the space – both theatrical and therapeutic. Facilitating clients to create the therapeutic space in order to enter their world creates some safety. He suggests we may go too quickly to the character before the transformation of the liminal/sacred space.

It has been a pleasure to write the Forward for this important book on 'Space, Place and Dramatherapy', a subject that has been neglected for too long. As an anthropologist, I am acutely aware of the importance of space, both actual and symbolic. The Temiars with whom I did my doctoral research had very clear spatial concepts which structure all individual and social lives: off the ground/ground; village/forest; river. This affected their behaviour in relation to these spaces, as well as the symbolism generated by the spaces in relation to their belief system (Jennings, 2006).

Prof Sue Jennings PhD
*Weston-Super-Mare UK and Penang Malaysia*

## Reference

Jennings, S. (2006) *Theatre, Ritual and Transformation: The Senoi Temiars.* Abingdon: Routledge.

# Preface

The importance of space and place is no new thing, having been debated and critiqued across multiple disciplines over the last 100 years including ethology, architecture, anthropology, human sciences, psychoanalysis, environmental psychology, cultural geography and the arts. A citation that I carry close to my practice is from the anthropologist Edward T. Hall who wrote that 'space is quintessentially a phenomenon that possesses the indisputable power to influence our emotional, sensorial and relational lives' (Hall, 1990). Before I was a dramatherapist, I worked as a performer, an art director, a scenographer, a visual artist and a producer, and Hall's words echoed throughout my professional life. So, when I became a dramatherapist, I was not surprised to find that the term *space* appeared ubiquitously across most arts and health publications. However, I was surprised to find that there was not one book dedicated to the critical enquiry of the many spaces that we can find in our discipline: creative, play, safe, ritual, liminal, encounter, imaginative ... to name a few. In my reading, I have come to the conclusion that space and place are concepts that have been overlooked and underwritten across the literature in arts and health and dramatherapy. In October 2013, author Toni Morrison Tweeted 'if there's a book that you want to read, but it hasn't been written yet, then you must write it' (Morrison, 2013). And so, we did.

This volume is important because, for the first time, questions of space and place in dramatherapy are gathered together and placed under the microscope, *under one roof*. This volume collates a range of dramatherapy practitioners from different backgrounds who, in their own way, present their readings of space and place in dramatherapy. I hope that this book will open up a dialogue of critical thinking about the many spaces and places among, between and with which we work. This book hopes to illuminate the importance of space and place, and I argue, through the existence of this volume, that space plays or should play explicitly a leading role in the dramatherapy discipline. Bringing together a collection of striking professionals and academics from around the world, this volume seeks to provide an innovative addition to the literature in the field of dramatherapy while opening up new avenues of thought, research, critical enquiry and practice.

Broadly speaking, it is in their inherent nature to connect humans to one another that the concepts of space and place give rise to a platform on which to share and collaborate together. The seed for this book was planted long ago, around 2014 when I began my dramatherapy training when my initial research into the dramatherapy therapeutic space sparked vigorous conversations between myself and colleagues, many of whom are in this volume, and bloomed during the Covid-19 pandemic. As I write this preface, the global pandemic continues to thrive, albeit more quietly since its first intrusion on the scene in early 2020, and in Paris, where I write from we have moved from spaces of fear, beyond exasperation and apathy. The French are even reintroducing the *la bise* (the kiss on the cheek, a typical French greeting) which disappeared from social life during the pandemic. We know full well that the coronavirus will not be the last of its kind to unsettle our known way of life, but what the Covid pandemic has shown us is that we are able to navigate the new and unknown psychological, relational and emotional territories of a collective-crisis and work within new physical and digital spaces all the while continuing to uphold the values and integrity of our discipline. To speak of the global coronavirus in the preface to this volume intends to situate this work in an important moment of human history and to illustrate how, with ever-increasing instability and disruption from pandemics, the global environmental crisis, recessions or war, the impact and importance of space and place have never before been so important to consider.

During the pandemic, many of us – if not all of us – questioned, rearranged or changed completely the spaces and places within which we work. Some dramatherapists chose to work from home via web links like Zoom or Teams and some chose to work outside and had to consider the implications of shifting from an indoor therapy space to an outdoor space on the therapeutic relationship (Bassingthwaighte, 2017). In our chapter, 'A Space of their Own: A case-study advocating appropriation of the domestic interior for well-being' (Sweeney and Messer, 2022), architect Sebastian Messer and I discuss one of my dramatherapy interventions during the first lockdown in Paris whereby through the online platform YouTube, I was able to maintain a therapeutic practice with children in precarious living circumstances. In the lead-up to this book, dramatherapist Ditty Dokter reflected upon the impact of working via online and digital platforms in her essay discussing the impact of Covid (Dokter, 2020), and in conversations with Ditty, she alluded to the potential of viewing screens as a play space and to the importance of considering embodiment within our online practices. She acknowledged that little has been published on this subject to date and while we were unable to provide more insight on this for this volume, it has sparked an ongoing and evolving debate about digital online dramatherapy.

In this book, Clive Holmwood noted that '[o]ur understanding of space is very much linked to our unique social and cultural understanding' (Holmwood, in this volume) and he reminds us that '[d]ifferent cultures have very different cultural understandings' of space which is vital to bear in mind. I acknowledge that while the title of this book suggests international perspectives, and while this volume did not set out to propose a particularly Euro-centric voice, there is a distinctively European thread running throughout. I believe that we need to hear from more varied voices across the globe on this essential and central subject if we are to have a fully fleshed out conversation and understanding of the impact of space and place in dramatherapy, a conversation that includes other voices and brings to the table complete diversity and inclusion. Writing an edited collection of chapters on space and place for the first time achieved what it could, and I am proud of all that we have achieved, but I hope that all voices feel welcome in this central discussion, and perhaps a second volume can achieve what this volume could not.

Preparing this book in the context of the global pandemic elucidated to me that more than ever, we need a place to come together, to close the gaps, to build bridges between countries, professionals and people. If we were not able to meet in person as we had done over many years as colleagues and friends, then we would meet through our art, our thoughts and our writing. While it was not its original intention, this book space became a place for meeting and connection, a place to reconnect and to play together again. Our hands could not hold one another but our words and thoughts could touch and throughout this process, and in reading our book, we get a sense of community and the presence of life. This book allowed me, if not all of us, to come out of isolation, to go out towards the world, and enter shared space. Without the shared space of collaboration that dramatherapy evokes, this book would not have been possible and I am eternally grateful to those who have joined me on this adventurous journey.

Eliza Sweeney

## References

Bassingthwaighte, L. (2017) 'Taking dramatherapy into the outside space', *Dramatherapy*, 38(1), pp. 16–31.

Dokter, D. (2020) 'Everybody in their boxes', *Dramatherapy Review*, 6(3), pp. 55–60.

Hall, E.T. (1990) *The Hidden Dimension*. New York: Anchor Books.

Morrison, T. (2013) *Twitter post*. Available at: https://twitter.com/tonimorrrison/status/395708227888771072?lang=en (Accessed 21 Jan 2022).

Sweeney, E. and Messer, S. (2022) 'A Space of Their Own: A Case-Study Advocating Appropriation of the Domestic Interior for Well-Being', in Scholze, J. *et al.* (eds.) *Interiors in the Era of COVID: Interior Design between the Public and Private Realms*. First edition. London [England]: Bloomsbury Visual Arts.

# Acknowledgements

I want to humbly thank everyone who has been a supporter of me on this journey and of this book project. I have the great fear that I am surely forgetting someone, and if I have, I apologize in advance. But you all know who you are, and this acknowledgement of thanks is to you.

I would like to express my deepest appreciation to the authors that you see named here today, without whom we would not have a book to read. Thank you for your time, patience and expertise, and for honouring me and this volume with your writing and thoughts and for trusting me with your experiences. I am truly humbled that you would join me on this adventure. I am indebted to Ellen Foynn Bruun, Helen Iles, Quy Gontran and Elsa El-Hachem who proofread the introduction and my own chapter. Thank you to Mary Putera for your endless wisdom and faith and for being a constant reminder of what it is to practise with integrity. Thank you to my PhD team, Rachel and Sebastian, who supported the idea that I keep this book project going alongside my research. Thank you, Alyson Coleman, for your warmthand encouragement to forge ahead in my academic pursuits. Thank you to the editorial team at Routledge Publishers who had faith in me and this project and who offered helpful guidance and support since day one.

To Phoebe, I am thankful for you and your endless curiosity and for being willing to build a fort or hut with me and play every day. Alex, I could not have undertaken this endeavour without you. Thank you for supporting my crazy idea to produce a book while starting a PhD, in the midst of a pandemic with a toddler and baby in tow. Your love, patience and encouragement have been a blessing.

Finally, I am very grateful to those of you who are reading this book. I hope that what you find here encourages reflection upon the different spaces within which you work and how they affect your practice and support those with whom you work. I am humbled that you took the time and gave space to our thoughts and I invite you to find a cosy nook, a warm place, a safe space and wish you happy reading.

# Prelude

## The Obviousness of Space of Anything But

*Eliza Sweeney*

I first encountered the use of a prelude in Marjin Niewenhuis and David Crouch's book *The Question of Space* (2017). They open with the proposition to begin with a prelude as opposed to a traditional introduction in order to warm up for the main event. In their case, the main event consists of a gathering of chapters that interrogate the notion of space as viewed through the lens of many interdisciplinary fields such as anthropology, performance and cultural geography. In the case of this book, I present a gathering of chapters that interrogate the notion of space and place through the lens of dramatherapy. Typically, we would expect to find an introduction in an academic text, a prologue in a novel and a prelude in a musical score, where all three are intent on foreshadowing the stories to come and providing a solid terrain from which these stories grow. The difference between prologue and prelude is that a prologue is comprised of *pro* (before) and *logos* (speech) means *before speech* whereas prelude is comprised of the prefix *pre* (before) and the Latin root *ledere* (play) meaning *before play* or *foreplay*. A prologue carries an essence of the intellectual whereas 'a prelude shares an ephemeral, esoteric and playful quality' (Nieuwenhuis and Crouch, 2017: xi). As drama and play therapist Sue Jennings has reminded us through her work on Neuro-Dramatic Play and Embodiment-Projection-Role, the lives of children begin pre-verbal, before speech and written language, and they communicate, learn and develop via the language of play. Play therefore precedes speech in human life. Whereas traditional psychotherapy techniques repose on the medium of speech and while speech is present in dramatherapy, dramatherapy is very often referred to as a non-verbal psychotherapy as it relies on its experiential, active, 'non-verbal' and playful approach for the most part. Therefore, if a book on dramatherapy is said to begin in any space or place, a playful one seems most appropriate. For a volume that addresses the subject of place and space in dramatherapy, a prelude finds its place in its 'foundational' nature 'in the same way as the key signature in a musical score anchors all thematic material and subsequent modulations' which is referred to as a 'preludial quality' (Fenner, 2011: 852). Writing this prelude was challenging as I strove to engage the prelude's playful nature in the toing and froing between anchoring the thematic material and balancing theory with anecdotal references

DOI: 10.4324/9781003252399-1

and practical examples. This book intends to offer a 'playground in which the meaning and experience of space [and place] can no longer be reduced to one single category or agency' (Nieuwenhuis and Crouch, 2017: xix) but expanded to involve multiple points of view and reflections which is recognized through the inclusion of a myriad of international voices and disciplines on the subject. As this prelude tries to demonstrate, the terms 'space' and 'place' may 'seem obvious to us' (Perec and Sturrock, 1997: 5) they are anything but, '[s]pace is no longer "this" or "that", dependent and confined to disciplinary knowledge, but instead becomes multiple, differential, personal, experiential and playful' (Nieuwenhuis and Crouch, 2017: xix).

## A Playful and Spatial Reading of S. Freud's Psychoanalytical Technique

When I wrote my first thesis in 2014, I stumbled upon a spatial reading of the therapeutic design of Sigmund Freud's psychoanalytical space with a particular focus on the Freudian couch, and I engaged with it to demonstrate how, since the early days of psychoanalytical thought, space has played a leading role in psychotherapeutic processes and methods in order to sustain my argument that the dramatherapy space can be considered in similar terms. The Freudian couch most specifically can be viewed as a stage space, a place where the inner life of the client is played out.

In 1913, when Freud spoke of the arrangement of the psychoanalytical space in The Psychoanalytic Technique (Freud, 1999), he presented his understanding of the importance of space in his attribution of a conscious and precise function to the couch-object within his office space. Freud proclaimed that the couch-object was not just an immutable object, going on to describe the specific function of the couch that was central to the success of the psychoanalytical process. Freud believed that the positioning of the couch prevented the contamination of transfer via the patient's associations by isolating the patient's body and thus withdrawing the transfer. Most recently Ogden (1985) and Celenza (2005) have viewed the couch as a 'potential space', capable of activating the dynamics of transference and countertransference and capable of maintaining safety and containing defence mechanisms which come back to Freud's original intention. It is also well known that Freud did not like to be looked at for eight hours a day but beyond this comfortable arrangement we can see that the placement of the couch in the space was intentional in order to affect the therapeutic process, and I argue that Freud's explicit decision to arrange the therapeutic space in such a particular and precise manner, with the conscious understanding of the spatial arrangement's effect on the therapeutic process, was a preliminary indicator as to the place of a spatial thinking in the psychotherapies and offers an opportunity for us to consider this in dramatherapy as well.

This perspective of the therapeutic psychoanalytical space has been taken up by numerous scholars and practitioners. French psychoanalyst and philosopher Jean Laplanche argues that 'space is the terrain where the singular problem of the patient is played out, where he is confronted by the existence, the permanence and the strength of his unconscious desires and fantasies' (Bourguignon, 1989: 137). Laplanche offers a topological reading of the psychoanalytical space wherein the arrangement of furniture elucidates the therapeutic relationship between the client and the therapist and supports the process of the psychoanalytical model. I reiterate Laplanche's point that the arrangement of the space impacts the therapeutic relationship and invites '*potential* action' (Hann, 2019: 28), but also that the orientation of the objects in space, or, in other terms, the arrangement of the space, invites or refuses particular behaviours, encounters and relationships. The conscious decision to arrange a space in such a precise manner lends Freud's design decisions to be considered as scenographic. Cultural scenography scholar Rachel Hann argues that 'scenographics are interventional acts of place orientation' where the 'staged acts' of placing furniture or objects are a precise way orients or focuses relationship, encounter or behaviour. I suggest that Freud's conscious decision to position the couch in such a particular way as to influence the therapeutic relationship was an undisputedly scenographic choice. Furthermore, Freud's aesthetic decision to adorn the couch with Turkish rugs and surround it with totems and visual art points to a distinctively scenographic trait where these aesthetic choices intended, whether consciously or unconsciously, to create a particular environment or atmosphere for the client. The couch with its Turkish rugs creates the perfect place for dreaming, similar to Aladdin's magic carpet, ready to whisk us away into story, to Ali Baba's cave of treasures. I propose that this atmosphere was created with the intention to support dreaming, storytelling and performance of an inner life and worlds. I therefore venture to suggest that in providing a space for reverie and dreaming, the Freudian couch becomes a stage space, an outer landscape where the inner story of the patient is *played out.*

In 1941, psychoanalyst Otto Fenichel offered his critique of the advantages of the Freudian couch in the analytical space remarking that the *ceremony* of entering a space that contains a couch and moving to lying down can produce a *magical* impression in the patient. He implies that the act of lying down creates the therapy space what I would call a heterotopia, a space out of time and space, which contributes to the process of regression. In a similar vein to Fenichel, Michael Fordham (1978) postulated that couch may facilitate regression by allowing them to more easily enter into deep thoughts or a dream state. This ritual or ceremony that Fenichel describes mirrors the dramatherapy process of shifting the client from the 'real world' into the play, stage or creative space of imagination and magical 'as ifs', where anything can happen. In dramatherapy, the client crosses one threshold when entering the room and again another when entering into the play or imaginative space of storytelling, role playing and improvisation, into a magical world of 'as ifs', creating Foucauldian heterotopia, *worlds within worlds* (1984). The ritual act of crossing over from one space to another contributes to the client's capacity to regress, find new meaning, express emotion and access the unconscious. In dramatherapy, our clients do not lie down on a couch but they do step into or onto a stage space, a playing space that is spatially defined by perhaps coloured scarves, curtains, room dividers or scotch tape on the floor. This is also a space, like on the Freudian couch, where their inner lives are *played out*.

Following this discussion of the Freudian couch as a scenographic, potential, ritual, dream space and a heterotopia, I contend that if such power can be wielded by objects and furniture arrangements, such as the stage-life phenomenon that the couch in the Freudian setting produces, then perhaps there is something to be said about our dramatherapy spaces, the way the space is designed, arranged, oriented as well as the aesthetic and atmosphere contribute to transference, relationship, dreaming and accessing inner lives. I wonder, where in dramatherapy is our 'couch'? Do the objects, design and layout of the room and the furniture within the drama therapy room have a potentially therapeutic function? Do they influence the therapeutic alliance between therapist and client? Answers to these questions as well as a reflection on whether these objects contribute to processes of creativity, containment, communication, emotion, psychology and behaviour are discussed in the body of this book.

## Space Is a Doubt

Before going any further, we should pause to reflect on what we are talking about and what we really want or mean to say when we use the terms 'space' and 'place' and whether it's really as important as the literature suggests. To truly understand the impact of space and place in dramatherapy and across history, it can be helpful to turn back to look at where we have come from as a discipline with regard to space and place. Turning back encourages us to look at the etymology of these words in order to offer a historical foundation for our contemporary use of them as well as looking back to the ways in which space and place have been engaged within our discipline to date. The idea of turning back was inspired by the post-structuralist and neo-Marxist movement the spatial turn, a movement that encapsulated a re-visiting and a re-thinking.

Enter the Roman God, Janus. According to legend, Janus was the god of time, of beginnings and endings, transitions and duality and he presided over passages, doorways and gates. He was present in transitional periods such as from war to peace, birth to death, journeys and other exchanges. Artistic representations of Janus most often depict him as having two faces that look in opposite directions: one looking forward towards the future and one looking back at the past. Janus reminds us of the importance of sometimes looking back to where we have come while (I hope) working forwards, passing through transitions, liminal spaces and thresholds towards the future.

Concepts, translations and uses of 'space' and 'place' have varied throughout recent history and are applied in multidisciplinary fields including geography, history, architecture, performance design, philosophy, anthropology, science, phenomenology, the arts and the arts therapies, to name a few. Returning to French novelist George Perec for a moment, Perec remarked that 'space becomes a question, ceases to be self-evident, ceases to be incorporated, ceases to be appropriated. Space is a doubt' (Perec and Sturrock, 1997: 91). This doubt sprouts from the uncertain etymological origins of our modern conceptions of 'space' and 'place' in relation to the ancient Greek translations of *chora* and *topos* as well as the cognate Latin *spatium* which is ubiquitously designated as the root for our modern understanding of *space*, intrinsically connected with notions of time. Circa 1200–1300, both place and space are cited etymologically as deriving from the Latin *spatium*, designating the dimensional extent of a room, a stretch of land or extension and generalizing any surface or volume while also meaning a stretch of time. While researching the etymology of these terms, I recalled some poetry that demonstrates this multiplicity of meaning and this temporal connection to space found within uses of the Old and Middle French word *espace* in sixteenth and seventeenth-century poetry. Ronsard's mid-sixteenth-century poem, 'Ode à Cassandre' gives an example of this, as he writes about the rose 'that in a short space' loses its beauty (Ronsard and Vaganay, 2014), while for Malherbe, in 'Consolation à du Périer' it lives 'only in the space of morning'.

Looking back to Ancient Greek, a complexity of synonyms for space existed: *chaos* as indefinite expanse, *topos* as limited expanse or occupied by a body, *meaxu* as an interval space, *meteoros* as an atmosphere, *chronos* as an expanse of time and finally *chora*. The *chora*, as described in Plato's *Timaeus*, is considered to be the metaphysical receptacle (*hupodochê*) through which the world comes to exist. Plato viewed space as a container, a grid or dimension within which matter and substance were contained but he alternated using the two terms *topos* (place) (τόπος) and *chóra* (space) (χώρα) interchangeably. Most commonly 'space' is considered to be the more abstract concept of the two terms, a belief that extends from Plato's writings in *Timaeus* that describes space as not having a relationship with its contents. Conversely to Plato's 'passive' viewpoint is Aristotle's 'active' view of space. Aristotle contended that all things that exist must exist somewhere, leading to theories of the natural 'place' of things, and because he used the term *(topos)* slightly more frequently, it became associated more frequently with place than space. For Aristotle, place and space are relational and he confirmed that all bodies contained within the receptacle (space) relate to the occupied vessel to which they pertain. Place therefore became relational which marked the first documented attempt (that I can find) at a coherent philosophy of space, with each text element (water, fire, earth, air) and substance (bodies, objects) being assigned a 'place' in *relationship* to the envelope of the corresponding body. Finally, because both Plato and Aristotle 'had recourse to concepts analogous to the modern English geographic place, as, respectively, *chora* and *topos*' (Agnew and Livingstone, 2011: 1), it is possible that the distinction between *chora* and *topos* as 'space' and 'place', respectively, throws doubt upon our modern translations of *chora* into *space* and *topos* into *place*. Aristotle's philosophies of active and relational space later trickled down to influence the thinking of Descartes, Kant, Hurssel, Merleau-Ponty, and Heidegger, to name a few modern philosophers whose ideas of our being in the world have driven much of contemporary thought about how we relate to the world and therefore, our environment, the spaces and places with and within which we exist. Specifically relevant to this volume is the work of Martin Heidegger, and while I cannot offer an expansive illustration of his thinking on space, being and time (Heidegger, 2002), it is worthy of note that he did propose that the way we inhabit the world and the way we are in our environment, on the face of the earth, is an extension of our identity, of who we are (ibid.), establishing the foundation for more contemporary discussions in environmental psychology about the influence of the built and natural environment on human life. Many of the chapters in this volume extend this thinking, directly or indirectly, and take time to reflect upon how the spaces of dramatherapy impact our being in the world with our clients, the therapeutic relationship, the client's individual sense of self, the group's identity or even the therapist's identity.

When considering how important space is, I took to the *Oxford English Dictionary* (Waite, 2012) only to discover that it dedicates approximately two pages to space and around three and a half to place. In 1966, anthropologist Edward T. Hall made reference to the number of times the word 'space' appeared in the Oxford English Dictionary noting that the word space took up '20% of all words' (Hall, 1990: 120). He noticed that what was more remarkable, beyond the statistical number of times that the word space shows up, was in fact the extent to which the term space is invested by humanity in a wide variety of areas of life: home, work, personal, public, social, psychological, geographical, etc. The frequency coupled with the ubiquity of application favours the view that 'space' as a concept holds an important place in our human (and arguably, other-than-human) lives. As the chapters in this book will demonstrate, there are a wide variety of views and interpretations regarding the meaning of space and place and how they are investigated in relation to drama therapy. Space and place are, most often, subjective. The book does not offer one final definition about what space and place are but rather invites the reader to consider all possibilities, concrete and abstract, containers and relationships, processes and theories and perhaps, one hopes, come to one's own conclusions about the importance of space and space in drama therapy.

## Conclusion

In the *Communication and the semantics of space*, Eliot Gaines proposes that 'we are not always aware of space and its capacity to alter the meaning of things' (Gaines, 2006: 179). Back in 2016 at my first dramatherapy conference in Romania for the European Federation of Dramatherapy, I presented my initial findings regarding the impact of space and spatial design on the therapeutic process. In Romania, Gaines' words rang true and I was surprised to witness how my presentation sparked some vigorous debate and discussion about space and dramatherapy with colleagues from which multiple meanings arose.

In one such discussion, a colleague divulged the disappointing reality that she once had to work in a repurposed sanitation closet because that was all that was available to her, and we spoke at length about the spaces within which we work, or are forced to work in, or are resigned to work in. It came to light that dramatherapists work in a myriad of spaces from repurposed meeting rooms to corridor spaces, classrooms, garden sheds, forests, living rooms and patient bedrooms. It became clearer as the conference went on that many dramatherapists just 'make do' with the spaces they are given because if they do not, the likely scenario to follow is that their sessions will not take place. This is not to say that dramatherapists are negligent and do not care for the rooms within which they work. On the contrary, I believe that dramatherapists are very much attuned to the spaces they work in, as this volume demonstrates, and many desire to have particular working spaces. Nevertheless, from observations and discussions with colleagues, I have come to realize that dramatherapists have become accustomed to being flexible, to working in not so perfect spaces, not so 'good enough' environments, so that their groups can happen, and while this flexibility may seem like a weakness, I'd argue that it can also be seen a strength in that in our flexibility we are able to access more clients in need. However, this strength becomes weakened when we do not explicitly reflect on and investigate the potentially powerful impact of these different spatial configurations on our clients each time we work in a new arena. As the pre-existing body of research and knowledge strongly suggests, space has an impact on human life, behaviour, culture, emotions, relationships and politics, which is a central argument to this book that '*where* things happen is critical to knowing *how* and *why* they happen' (Warf and Arias, 2014). Even if we cannot make decisions about *where* we practice, we can reflect clinically and critically about the ways in which the room we work within is arranged, designed or furnished in order to provide the best 'good enough' environment for our clients. Over time, I began to question how our clients must feel in a particular space and what meaning it could hold for them. I wondered what the space within which we work was communicating to them about the importance of their illness or personal challenges; I wondered what message was being sent. Architects Charles Jencks and Edwin Heathcote wrote, in 'The Architecture of Hope: Maggie's Cancer Caring Centres', that architecture sends clear messages: 'you matter, your feelings are important to us, to society' (Jencks and Heathcote, 2015: 41–42) and the environment within which we work will either increase or decrease the value and quality of these messages. Similar thought is espoused by environmental psychologists who argue that the built and natural environments have an effect on human development, relationships and health. The field of environmental psychology has demonstrated that the way a room is designed, the colours and fabrics that are chosen, the temperature, air flow and quality of the space, the access to nature, the lighting and a host of other criteria will influence and impact human health and well-being. During the last 50 years, there has been vigorous growth in studies concerned with human-to-environment relations. Investigations in human ethology, social and environmental psychology

(Kearns and Gesler, 1998; Shepley and Danko, 2017; Wells and Donofrio, 2011), sociology, human geography (Adams-Hutcheson, 2017; Agnew and Livingstone, 2011; Pini, Dhavernas and Gibson, 2019), anthropology, urban planning, environmental design and architecture traditions demonstrate this. The influence of space on health and development has been extensively argued in various fields including cultural geography, anthropology and the newly evolved field of environmental psychology. These studies demonstrate that different spaces demand different relationships and, by consequence, provoke distinct spatial, sensorial, affective and mental experiences. A space that is enclosed, without natural lighting, and full of accessories, furniture and objects will, for example, create a very different ambiance and experience than an open, light, well-organized and considered space. Anthropologist Edward T. Hall once wrote that 'practically everything that man is, is associated with space (…) man and his environment participate in the formation of one another' (Hall, 1990: 95) and Winston Churchill is also renowned for having said something similar along the lines of, we shape our buildings and in turn they shape us. Furthermore, environmental psychologists Bell, Fisher, Baum, and Greene suggest that 'relations between the behaviour and experience of an individual and their physical space or environment' (Bell, 2001: 167) must be understood in order to understand *how* the environment impacts human life and well-being which informs *how* we can work *with* space and the environment to support behaviour, relations, experiences, well-being. As I sit and read the literature on environmental psychology and tune into the stories of colleagues working in such varied, and occasionally desperate spaces, the concern about what message is being communicated to our clients is overshadowed by a louder question: what are these spaces *doing* and how can we understand what they are doing so that we can offer best practice?

What often strikes me is that '[d]rama therapy theory has mainly focused on concepts such as distance (Landy, 1983; Scheff, 1979), roles (Johnson, 1982; Landy, 1991, 1992), performance (Emunah and Johnson, 1983) and other aspects that are common to theatre/drama and therapy' but 'the role of the stage as an element that affects the drama therapy process rarely has been taken into account' (Pendzik, 1994: 25). More recently, art therapy scholar Patricia Fenner has also acknowledged this absence of reflection on space in the arts therapies remarking how 'the physical setting within which therapy takes place has attracted little research attention to date' (Fenner, 2011: 852). Dramatherapist Joanna Jaaniste notes that across the mountain of dramatherapy literature available, 'there is a significantly higher ratio of reference to ritual in comparison with the space or place where it happens' (Jaaniste in this volume), reiterating just one of the many ways in which the notion of space has remained peripheral to our discipline. Across wider studies in theatre and drama, we can find evidence of reflections on the importance of space. One example where we can see beginnings of spatial thinking in dramatherapy is through the appropriation of theatre scholar Richard Schechner's work with actors on rasaesthetics for dramatherapy purposes. The Rasa Boxes technique has a distinctively spatially driven methodology, where responses to emotions can be drawn, written or moved through space, advocating for an acknowledgement that emotional experiences can be influenced by space. Schechner defines rasa as an emotional or aesthetic response that 'fills space, joining the outside to the inside, what was outside is transformed into what is inside' (Schechner, 2001: 29). Schechner's theories of space extend to his reflections on environmental theatre design where he proposes that *sense-making* comes from a specific relationship to space, 'from *within* the spaces of the *body* to *within* the spaces of the *place* being explored' (Schechner, 1971: 388). He has an explicit alignment with theories espoused by environmental psychologists who understand the power of space to affect. I interpret Schechner's positioning as an invitation to explore with deep curiosity the spaces within which we work, to be open to the ways in which space encourages action, relationship, movement, emotion and change, and to listen to what space has to say (Schechner, 1968).

Of course, this book does not seek to claim that reflections and discussions on the subject of space have been entirely neglected by our discipline and recognizes many examples of moments over time where space was becoming a central focus point. There are some texts that speak directly to particular spaces within the context of a wider methodology or focus, such as Salvo Pitruzzella's book 'Drama, Creativity and Intersubjectivity: The Roots of Change in Dramatherapy' (Pitruzzella, 2017), Phil Jones' devotion to the 'play space' (Jones, 1996), David Read Johnson's writings on the 'playspace' (one word) in Developmental Transformations, to name a few and I acknowledge there are many more, however, while they speak *to* space, the focus is not specifically *on* space, where space is considered as playing a leading role. Susana Pendzik's 1994 publication, *The theatre stage and the sacred space: a comparison* (Pendzik, 1994) is one example where a dramatherapist does put space and place under the spotlight and it is a welcomed read. Over the past 20 years, humanistic art therapies have also gently discussed the therapeutic qualities of the art therapy studio (Fenner, 2011; Ings, 2014; Knill, Levine and Levine, 2005; McNiff, 2004), thoughts which contribute to a deeper reflection on the potentially therapeutic effects of the environment. Notably, in his article '*Keeping the Studio*', Shaun McNiff draws our attention to the studio space as a 'therapeutic community' that provides 'atmospheric medicines' (McNiff, 1995) as a medium for change and Patricia Fenner further this idea in her paper *'Place, matter and meaning: extending the relationship in the psychotherapies'* evoking ideas about how the surrounding environment plays a leading role. She states, '[h]istorically the content of these psychological exchanges has been the focus of interest with only fleeting consideration given to where they are taking place and how these environments might play a role in the nature, tone and content of those intimate encounters' (Fenner, 2011: 851). Furthermore, Anna Chesner is cited as discussing the necessity of the therapeutic space in the following terms:

The dramatherapeutic experience invites the taking of risks. Clients are invited to journey together into the unknown. It is a matter of respect for the element of risk involved in this process that the boundaries of the therapeutic space need to be establish and honoured.

(Jennings, 1994: 59)

Chesner and Jennings have explored methodologies and practical implications of ensuring a safe space for clients, which centre upon the rules of the session, noting that the space needs to be private, without interruption, at the same time each week, and advocating that a dedicated dramatherapy space is the best possible solution. In this volume, Amanda Musicka-Williams outlines the essential factors that assist in the co-creation of a dramatherapy space in an educational setting. Altogether, Fenner, Chesner, Schechner, Pitruzzella, Johnson, Pendzik, Jennings, McNiff and others, I am sure, reinforce Warf and Arias' argument that *where* therapy occurs impacts *what* occurs but their innovative thoughts and reflections are scattered across multiple publications. Centralizing the discussion on space and place puts it at the heart of the matter, under the spotlight, to play the leading role.

As mentioned above, sometimes looking back to where we have come from is required in order to move forward. This introductory chapter has taken a look back to the etymology of the terms 'space' and 'place', simplifying a much more complex argument that I could do justice to here. It has also reflected upon instances in history where space and psychotherapy have joined forces and worked together to bolster the therapeutic process, as seen through Freud's couch. It has reflected on the timeliness of this book, during a global pandemic, as a meeting place for practitioners to come together in a shared space and the need we all share to have collective spaces once more and I have tried to spark debate about the importance of spatial design in dramatherapy. Framing this introduction with the 'spatial turn' required retrospection, a looking back, but it also signifies a change in direction. Dramatherapy is, I would argue, a relatively constant discipline with regard to the founding rituals, methods, techniques and methodologies that are applied and continue to be used in most drama therapy cultures, that I know of. I am most specialized in European cultures and speak through this lens. Invoking the notion of a spatial turn throughout this drama therapy book is intended as a provocation to the discipline to change directions and consider other ways of doing dramatherapy, to go *beyond dramatherapy*. Through cultural scenographer and scholar Rachel Hann's book 'Beyond Scenography' (2019), I was introduced to the work of cultural theorist Homi Bhabha's with regard to this term, *the beyond*. Hann states that

Homi Bhabha outlines how the term 'signifies spatial distance, marks progress, promises the future; but our imitations of exceeding the barrier or boundary – the very act of going beyond – are unknowable, unrepresentable, without a return to the "present" which, in the process of repetition, becomes disjunct and displaced'.

(Hann, 2019: 1)

Moving from scenographic, architectural and sound spaces through to educational, play, ritual and spiritual spaces of dramatherapy practice, this book proposes a focus on present dramatherapy practice as presented through the multitude of case studies and perspectives offered within its pages. As this volume attests, space is not always physical, and there are relational spaces, ritual spaces and intersubjective spaces that also require navigation and exploration.

In the words of poet Pierre Albert Birot, 'At the door of the house who will come knocking? An open door, we enter; A closed door, a den; The world's pulse beats beyond my door' (Bachelard and Jolas, 2014). As the first book dedicated entirely to space, place and dramatherapy, this book is an opening of doors or windows in some respect. This book was formed in such a way that it invites you to spend time in each space in quiet reflection and invites you to take the time to think about your own practice, past, present or future, and how space informs or affects you, the process and the participants in dramatherapy as well as in wider practices of arts and health. It is this volume's intention and hope that by viewing present practice through a spatial lens, we might be encouraged even inspired to go *beyond* current ways of practicing, thinking and theorizing dramatherapy into new spaces and places of practice.

## References

Adams-Hutcheson, G. (2017) 'Spatialising skin: Pushing the boundaries of trauma geographies', *Emotion, Space and Society*, 24, pp. 105–112. Available at: 10.1016/j.emospa.2016.03.002

Agnew, J.A. and Livingstone, D.N. (eds.) (2011) *The SAGE Handbook of Geographical Knowledge*. Los Angeles: SAGE.

Bachelard, G. and Jolas, M. (2014) *The Poetics of Space*. New edition. New York, NY: Penguin Books (Penguin classics).

Bell, P.A. (ed.) (2001) *Environmental Psychology*. 5th ed. Fort Worth, TX: Harcourt College Publishers [u.a.].

Bourguignon, A. (ed.) (1989) *Traduire Freud*. 1st ed. Paris: Presses Universitaires de France.

Celenza, A. (2005). Vis-à-vis the couch: Where is the psychoanalysis. *International Journal of Psychoanalysis*, 86, pp. 1645–1659. Available at: 10.1516/5R0C-T87T-CK9D-86UJ

Emunah, R., and Johnson, D.R. (1983). 'The impact of theatrical performance on the self-images of psychiatric patients'. *The Arts in Psychotherapy*, 10, pp.233–239.

Fenner, P. (2011) 'Place, matter and meaning: Extending the relationship in psychological therapies', *Health & Place*, 17(3), pp. 851–857. Available at: 10.1016/j.healthplace.2011.03.011

Freud, S. (1999) *The Standard Edition of the Complete Psychological Works of Sigmund Freud*. Repr. Edited by J. Strachey. London: Hogarth Press.

Fordham, M. (1978/2018). *Jungian Psychotherapy. A Study in Analytical Psychology*. New York: Routledge.

Gaines, E. (2006) 'Communication and the semiotics of space', *Journal of Creative Communications*, 1(2), pp. 173–181. Available at: 10.1177/097325860600100203

Hall, E.T. (1990) *The Hidden Dimension*. New York, NY: Anchor Books.

Hann, R. (2019) *Beyond Scenography*. New York, NY: Routledge, Taylor & Francis Group.

Heidegger, M. (2002) *Being and Time*. Reprint. Malden, MA: Blackwell.

Ings, W. (2014) 'Embodied drawing: A case study in narrative design', *Artifact*, 3(2), pp. 2.1–2.10.

Jencks, C. and Heathcote, E. (2015) *The Architecture of Hope: Maggie's Cancer Caring Centres*. London: Frances Lincoln.

Jennings, S. (ed.) (1994) *The Handbook of Dramatherapy*. London; New York: Routledge.

Jones, P. (1996) *Drama as Therapy: Theatre as Living*. London; New York: Routledge.

Johnson (1982). 'Developmental approaches in drama therapy', *The Arts in Psychotherapy*, 9(3), pp. 183–189. Available at: 10.1016/0197-4556(82)90035-1

Kearns, R.A. and Gesler, W.M. (eds.) (1998) *Putting Health into Place: Landscape, Identity, and Well-Being*. 1st ed. Syracuse, NY: Syracuse University Press (Space, place, and society).

Knill, P.J., Levine, E.G. and Levine, S.K. (2005) *Principles and Practice of Expressive Arts Therapy: Toward a Therapeutic Aesthetics*. London; Philadelphia: Jessica Kingsley Publishers.

Landy, R.J. (1983). 'The use of distancing in drama therapy'. *The Arts in Psychotherapy*, 10(3), pp. 175–185. Available at: 10.1016/0197-4556(83)90006-0.

Landy, R.J. (1991). 'The drama therapy role method', Dramatherapy, 14(2), pp. 7–15. Available at: 10.1080/02630672.1992.9689810

Landy (1992). 'The drama therapy role method', *Dramatherapy*, 14(2), pp. 7–15.

McNiff, S. (1995) 'Keeping the studio', *Art Therapy*, 12(3), pp. 179–183. Available at: 10.1080/07421656.1995.10759156

McNiff, S. (2004) *Art Heals: How Creativity Cures the Soul*. Boston: Shambhala.

Nieuwenhuis, M. and Crouch, D. (eds.) (2017) *The Question of Space: Interrogating the Spatial Turn between Disciplines*. London; New York: Rowman & Littlefield International, Ltd (Place, memory, affect).

Ogden, T. (1985). 'On potential space'. '*International Journal of Psychoanalysis*, 66, pp. 129–141.

Pendzik, S. (1994) 'The theatre stage and the sacred space: A comparison', *The Arts in Psychotherapy*, 21(1), pp. 25–35. Available at: 10.1016/0197-4556(94)90034-5

Perec, G. and Sturrock, J. (1997) *Species of Spaces and Other Pieces*. London; New York, NY: Penguin Books (Penguin twentieth-century classics).

Pini, B., Dhavernas, C. and Gibson, M. (2019) 'The emotional geographies of the "livingdying"', *Emotion, Space and Society*, 33, p. 100624. Available at: 10.1016/j.emospa.2019.100624

Pitruzzella, S. (2017) *Drama, Creativity, and Intersubjectivity: The Roots of Change in Dramatherapy*. London: Routledge, Taylor & Francis Group.

Ronsard, P. de and Vaganay, H. (2014) *Les Odes: Texte de 1578*. Paris: Éditions Classiques Garnier numérique.

Schechner, R. (1968) '6 axioms for environmental theatre', *The Drama Review: TDR*, 12(3), p. 41. Available at: 10.2307/1144353

Schechner, R. (1971) 'On environmental design', *Educational Theatre Journal*, 23(4), p. 379. Available at: 10.2307/3205747

Schechner, R. (2001) 'Rasaesthetics', *TDR/The Drama Review*, 45(3), pp. 27–50. Available at: 10.1162/10542040152587105

Scheff, T.J. (1979). *Catharsis in Healing, Ritual, and Drama / T. J. Scheff*. Berkeley: University of California Press.

Shepley, M.M. and Danko, S. (2017) 'Design as healing: The next generation of research-informed practice: Design as healing', *Journal of Interior Design*, 42(1), pp. 5–7. Available at: 10.1111/joid.12090

Waite, M. (ed.) (2012) *Paperback Oxford English Dictionary*. 7th ed. Oxford: Oxford University Press.

Warf, B. and Arias, S. (eds.) (2014) *The Spatial Turn: Interdisciplinary Perspectives*. 1. issued in paperback. London: Routledge (Routledge studies in human geography, 26).

Wells, N.M. and Donofrio, G.A. (2011) 'Urban Planning, the Natural Environment, and Public Health', in *Encyclopedia of Environmental Health*. Elsevier, pp. 565–575. Available at: 10.1016/B978-0-444-52272-6.00480-3

Part 1

# The Built Environment and Scenography in Dramatherapy

*Eliza Sweeney*

# 1 Teachings from Echo

*Ellen Foyn Bruun*

## Introduction

In dramatherapy, we listen with all our senses and aim to tune into others, to the world and to ourselves. We may experience that the without and within dissolve and become blurred. What is the space that holds us together? What is the space that separates us? In this chapter, I want to raise awareness of how we can enable clients and ourselves to tune in to the human body's urge for poetic sense-making of complex phenomena such as within and without. I am interested in investigating how our awareness of being in space and being space may be explored in dramatherapy supported with inspiration from voicework. When we work with myths and stories we may be surprised and become connected to their archetypal energies. This may trigger our personal complexes and in turn, allow us to explore these within the containing space of the dramatherapy session. The myth of Echo has fascinated me for years and some years ago I got a chance to explore it in a dramatherapy context that aimed to allow for an experiential process of connecting to deep embodied knowing of echoes within and without. In this chapter, I will investigate how we can better understand and frame these kinds of experiential reverberations.

The kind of space I propose stems from my interest in the interface of dramatherapy and voicework. It suggests an understanding of space as a process rather than as something fixed. The notion of space here is experiential and emergent. It resonates with the potential space of play and art making, as coined by Donald W. Winnicott (1971). In the play space, we explore our inner and outer worlds through embodied creative imagination. Anything can happen here, or can it? I wonder. Stephen K. Levine (1997: 28) asks, under what conditions does artistic expression become therapeutic and this also leads to wondering the opposite. Through our creative imagination and skills, we can retell or transform our experiences, again and again. At the origin of this, is the act of *Poiesis*, as originally introduced by Aristotle (Levine, 2009: 30). For the discussion here, I want to explore space not only as metaphor but also as material phenomenon relating to our being with ourselves, others and the world. To frame this notion of space I will draw on the phenomenology of perception as introduced by Maurice Merleau-Ponty (2012: 205) asserting

DOI: 10.4324/9781003252399-3

that we 'have no other means of knowing the human body that by living it, that is taking up for myself the drama that moves through it and by merging with it'. This means that 'I am my body' (Merleau-Ponty, 2012: 151) as a subjective lived experience, rather than having a body. I will also look into how Gaston Bachelard (2014) offers a phenomenological thinking that embeds space not only in the imaginative but also offers an onto-epistemic understanding of space for dramatherapy processes.

The chapter places emphasis on imagination and poetic meaning-making. These two concepts resonate with Levine's claim (2009: 25) that arts therapies ultimately rest on *Poiesis,* our capacity to respond and change the world through the act of shaping what is given to us. Levine asserts that the 'play of imagination must be placed at the center of the human capacity for shaping it we are to understand this power in its own right' (Knill, Levine and Levine, 2005: 11). He also reminds us that the senses not only give us bodily impressions, but they also make sense and indicate where to act (Levine and Moon, 2019: 5). This resonates well with Bachelard and the practice I propose in this chapter with the Echo workshop, which may provide experiential recognition of emergent spaces within and without through the integration of somatic awareness and imagination. With a focus on careful listening (Bruun, 2015) that engages all the senses, the dramatherapy space is understood here as a place for *Poiesis* to unfold experientially in motion, dynamic and transformative.

## The World of the Body

In drama and theatre-based practice, the subjective body is also the object, in terms of what is being shaped. The body is the vehicle, and the emphasis is on its capacity to stage itself. The subjective body is explored as access *to* the world, while at the same time being in interaction with itself *as* world, thus reiterating the phenomenology of the body that underscores the body as lived experience. Merleau-Ponty (2012: 84) underpins that the 'body is the vehicle of being in the world and, for a living being, having a body means being united with a definite milieu, merging with certain projects, and being perpetually engaged therein'. The body subject not only creates but is created in a historical, cultural and situated world. It is actively shaping itself and at the same time shaped by the world it is in. How we shape ourselves depends deeply on our life circumstances, upbringing and other people's thoughts and actions. The innate potential of our biological body is activated depending on lived experience, for better or worse. This activation happens through all kinds of experiences, including drama. It is no wonder that drama is commonly understood as training for life because when we explore ourselves through role, improvisation or enactment, we are subject-object doubled up, in the play space as the me *and* not-me. In play, and framed in symbolic reality, the belief is that the subject will be allowed to deepen its lived experience as world while gaining access to more of its own world, inner and outer. In the aesthetic exploration, the body-subject can experience itself as subject-object, by using lived experience while creating new lived experience. To achieve this, we, as dramatherapists, train our imaginative capacity to be able to be fully engaged in play while at the same time, remaining outside of it. The concepts of over-distance and under-distance, introduced by Robert Landy (1994), are useful in this regard. As for actors on stage, best performance happens when we are fully present, body and mind.

In the article with the significant title, 'The space that divides and connects. Betweenness and the intersubjective perspective', Salvo Pitruzzella (2018) elaborates on how intersubjectivity is part of our nature and the foundation for our relational capacity. The subjective body is touched by the world, both materially and as something bigger than the material. This agrees with Merleau-Ponty's dialectical understanding of lived experience as entailing and intertwining the totality of the individual's subjectivity and intersubjectivity (Low, 1992). In dramatherapy we want to provide the opportunity to connect to the transpersonal realm of intersubjectivity because this is where our individuality deepens and expands, and where we can land in another kind of space and feeling of belonging. We can meet through metaphor and story, in the arts and poetry, because in that space we have the opportunity to project our subjective world in symbolic form, and create aesthetic distance and recognition. This also resonates with the basic model for dramatherapy, introduced by Sue Jennings, based on the infant's development from embodiment to projection to role, known as the EPR-model (Jennings, 1994, Langley, 2006).

## Bachelard's Philosophy of Space and Dramatherapy

Bachelard's hermeneutics of space, or topoanalysis, is part of his interest in analysing the poetic works of imagination. In the introduction to *The Poetics of Space*, Bachelard (2014: 1) writes, 'the philosophy of poetry must acknowledge that the poetic has no past, at least no recent past, in which its preparation and appearance could be followed'. This means that the poetic image is original, it is born and given life in the here-and-now moment. Similarly, in dramatherapy, change and healing occur through the immediate life-giving force of the artistic creation through *Poiesis*. Bachelard (2014: 6) introduces daydreaming or reverie as a kind of logic determined by intuition and embodied listening. For him, poetic imagination stems from this kind of pre-linguistic and embodied logos, and, in my view, this is the kind of experiential way of knowing that we invite in dramatherapy and the arts in general. When I introduce the exploration of the myth of Echo, I will clarify this further and illuminate the way in which it has bearing for drama and the arts as therapy and, as a way of knowing. When we recognize the autonomy of the poetic image, it means that the non-sense, may have sense.

Bachelard understands daydreaming as a healthy way in which individuals self-regulate and process inner and outer experience. In daydreaming the individual meets the poetic image with immediate awareness in a way that also reverberates within and without the body, as unique experiential phenomenon on a transpersonal level (Bachelard, 2014: 4). Similarly, in dramatherapy, Pitruzzella (2013) investigates poet William Blake's imagination in connection with inner listening and reverie as a source for healthy development. Pitruzzella writes that '[i]magination needs the material provided by the Inner Listening; it needs to be in contact with the richness of our world of emotions, feelings and stories, to remain not a mere fantasy, which goes in the direction of denying the world, rather than being a tool to meet it' (Pitruzzella, 2013: 83). Imbricated in this is an important onto-epistemic claim and wisdom that resonates with Bachelard. It is also related to the question I posed earlier with Levine (1997: 28) about the conditions necessary for artistic expression to become therapeutic as opposed to a mere reactive acting out. Pitruzzella's thinking resonates with the notion of the *intelligence of feeling* introduced by Robert Witkin (1974) that distinguishes between subjective-reactive and subjective-reflexive actions. Based on this, British arts educator Malcolm Ross explains that at the heart of art as a way of knowing is the subject-reflexive action as 'an account of creativity [in the arts] that prioritized the feeling of inter-action between the individual student's unique formative intuitions and the medium they were working in' (Ross, 2013: 14). This describes well what Pitruzzella refers to as inner listening that has to do with embodied and sensate feeling intelligence. When we work with making form from an inner, felt intention, we process our life experiences. In line with Pitruzzella, the kind of imagination we want to foster and stimulate in dramatherapy is this kind of reflexive and healthy creativity that deals with the world and enables us to do so, with all its suffering, pain and discomfort. As I see it, Bachelard's notion of imagination as space epitomizes a similar experience, namely that of meeting the poetic image as phenomenon on its own, as a surprise that hits immediately the core of our being, our soul. Space here, therefore, is presented as somatic and understood as subjective lived experience including the transpersonal. It is embodied and metaphorical and the place for *Poiesis*, our ability to dwell in imagination as an autonomous space. This space recalls Winnicott's (1971) potential space, that place where the infant and later the adult, connects inner and outer realities through play, imagination and the arts.

## Why Echo?

One of the great Greek myths, Echo presents the tragic tale of a young nymph. According to Ovid's *Metamorphoses* (Liveley, 2011), Echo was a beautiful nymph whose one failing was that she was fond of talking and always would have the last word. In Ovid's version, she is a loquacious nymph, 'capable of entertaining people with long-winded discourses [*sermones*]' (Cavarero, 2005: 165). When Juno discovers that Echo has helped the nymphs escape after they had fornicated with her husband Jupiter, she curses her. After Juno's curse, Echo is condemned to a life where she can only repeat what she hears. She thereby has no control of her speech. She may only react after someone has spoken and can only repeat the last sound uttered by the other. Echo, in this way, remains pure voice and vocal resonance, since the logical meaning of the words gets distorted (Cavarero, 2005: 168). Echo is commonly viewed negatively due to her dependent position, where the act of responding is not owned by her. With no identity or agency of her own, Echo and the act of echoing do not represent qualities we usually approve of in Western society.

And yet, I was drawn to Echo. I was drawn towards her femininity, her status as nymph, not Goddess, and my intuitive assumption was that it would be worth-while investigating her fate, if not only to challenge the negative assumptions. During my dramatherapy training, I came across Patricia Berry's (1982) *Echo's subtle body: Contribution to an archetypal psychology*. Echo's fate of being silenced by Juno and condemned only to imitation, reminded me of my earlier French literary studies of Honoré de Balzac's (1845) *The unknown masterpiece (Le Chef-d'oeuvre Inconnu)*, a philosophical short story reverberating with several muted female figures from Pygmalion's model Galatea and the three Marys to the naked young woman in the artist's atelier (Bruun, 1981). Balzac's complex short story discusses the purpose of art and artists based on the video-centric ideal of Western art history. Seeing, for the male artists here, is associated with conquering. At a closer reading, the muted female voices emerge with *La belle noiseuse*, as a common figure for what the artist really needs to 'see' to create. 'Noiseuse' refers to noise and sensory listening, beyond the direct seeing with the eyes (Bruun, 1981). Maybe hiking in the Norwegian mountains as a child was also part of my intuitive feeling of sisterhood with Echo. What joy and pleasure it was to shout out and get the sounds in return – resounding throughout in the landscape.

Then, for well over a decade, I was lucky to co-facilitate a series of workshops with emphasis on voicework in dramatherapy with my partner, David Keir Wright (1943–2020). The integration of the Roy Hart approach to voicework with dramatherapy was our focus (Bruun and Wright, 2013, Bruun, 2015). South African actor Roy Hart (1926–1975) was the pupil of Alfred Wolfsohn (1896–1962). They represent two generations of pioneering voicework throughout the twentieth century that still hold prominent importance today through The Roy Hart International Arts Centre in the South of France (*Centre Artistique Internationale Roy Hart*). As a foundation for this voice pedagogy is Wolfsohn's notion of 'the unchained voice' based on his self-healing of traumatic, aural hallucinations after the First World War (Baker and Uhlig, 2011: 27). Wolfsohn understood the voice as the mirror of the soul (Pikes, 2019: 32). He was inspired by Jungian thinking and the transpersonal imaginative legacy of the archetypes as a pool for investigating and expanding the individual's many voices. The Wolfsohn/Hart legacy offers opportunities to explore these many vocal selves, as an expanded vocal repertoire with emphasis on sounding without 'restrictions' often with the only intention of exploring how breath, movement and making vocal sounds may inspire one another mutually. This kind of messy voicework resonates with Echo's babble and distortion of meaning of the message received. Vocal imagination may surface from unknown subjective and intersubjective realms, felt throughout the physical body as resonance.

The emphasis on voice deepened my understanding of dramatherapy because it brought me closer to the physical body, much like the actor/player, re-inventing herself through deepening the listening inwards and revitalizing silenced and hidden parts, stories and experiences (Bruun, 2015). I realized, not only intuitively but also theoretically, the depth of Pitruzzella's (2013) investigation of imagination and play, based in *Poiesis* as a performative act in line with Bachelard's insistence of the autonomy of the poetic image. Exploratory voicework such as the legacy from Wolfsohn/Hart is on the same wavelength as the kind of process that Bachelard encourages through daydreaming and reverie inviting the poetic image to surface from the unconscious 'in its newness [that] opens a future to language' (Bachelard and Gaudin, 1987). One specifically helpful factor was the experiential awareness of voicework being anchored so fundamentally of the physicality of breath. This simple fact epitomizes that voicework is two-fold. On the one hand, it is about vocal production, directed outwards, as communication. This includes how we use our voice to explore vocal range and possibilities when sounding, singing and speaking, on stage, as public speakers, on stage or in life in general. On the other hand, voicework is about listening and receptive attention, directed inwards (Bruun, 2015). This includes tuning into somatic processes of all kinds; how we are silent and aware of silence; how we are present and attuned to the totality of our subjectivity, to other living beings, to ourselves and to the planet. Awareness of breath and breathing can be stimulated in many ways. For me, a shift of awareness happened when I was introduced to voice teacher Catherine Fitzmaurice (2015) and her explicit purpose of releasing the breathing reflex and sensitizing somatic awareness of vocal sounding (Bruun, 2021).

As in play and drama, the core of voicework might be pinned down to the oscillation of introversion and extroversion in the fluid state of being and becoming (Bruun, 2015). My point here is that our imagination stems from how we function physically. What reverberates as poetic imagination throughout our bodies is material and, as Bachelard claims, autonomous and intersubjective. This is also how I understand Pitruzzella's (2013: 83) concept of Inner Listening that also draws attention to embodied *aural* perception and takes us closer to Echo. It is opposed to *visual* perception, as represented in the story by Narcissus. According to feminist philosopher Adriana Cavarero (2005), there is a dominant understanding in Western philosophy to favour visuality over aurality, image over sound, as in speech over voice, semantics over phonetics and writing over oral speaking. Cavarero (2005) is critical to the way the logo-centric mind-over-body tradition of Western philosophy uncritically disregards sounding and privileges semantics over sound. She puts emphasis on the autonomy of sound and resonance and, for her, Echo represents a counter-narrative of Western philosophy. This claim only strengthened my desire to explore the story of Echo in a dramatherapy context. Both Berry (1982: 118) and Cavarero (2005: 168) make a point of how Echo's responses distort language and empty its meaning through repetition. Rather than repeating the words, Echo repeats their sounds. Without a choice, she simply yields to the physical phenomenon of the echo, imitating even the timbre of the voice. By this, the autonomy of sound and sounding comes to the foreground.

### The Echo Workshop

The opportunity to investigate the story of Echo experientially arrived in 2016 at the 2nd European Federation of Dramatherapy Conference, *Opening the Curtains,* in Bucharest, Romania (*European Federation of Dramatherapy*). My co-facilitator, Wright and I prepared a workshop where we brought together voice and dramatherapy practice, based on our shared insights and curiosities. At the centre of the two-hour session, 'Voices from within and without – Echoes from nature', was the story of Echo from Ovid's *Metamorphoses* (Liveley, 2011). I will not analyse what happened during the workshop that was attended by around twenty-five conference participants. What is relevant here is the intention and thinking behind the workshop as a poetic space inviting the participants to explore experientially subjective and intersubjective echoes within and without. The rationale of the experiential offerings during the workshop was to welcome the embodied imagination as an autonomous place of poetic encounter through the performative practice. Echoing was emphasized as complex and multidimensional practice throughout the workshop and reflected as theme in Ovid's text and William Wordsworth's (2018) poem: *Yes, it was the mountain echo.*

The intention for introducing Wordsworth's poem in addition to the story itself was to open some broader perspectives on the theme than the notion of Echo's vocal imitation and repetition as 'negative'. Conversely, Wordsworth's (2018) poem promotes the positive act of echoing suggesting also the autonomy of the aural reflection, as: 'Like – but Oh, how different'. What is our connection as humans to this space of Echo's body-less voice? Can we hear this reactive calling from within our own nature? How do we relate to this receptive, intuitive or 'unconscious', internal echo within? These were questions we asked ourselves in the planning of the workshop. Being present in each moment of our own lives is a challenge in the world today. Being receptive with an open non-judgmental mind requires that we develop sensitivity to the inner voices and the echoes from our own nature and instinctual yearning for healthy self-regulation – listening to the voice of nature, rebounding off the rocks, our bones maybe.

The workshop was carefully designed in six stages: focus, warm-up, bridge-in, main event, bridge-out and grounding – the intention being that each exercise would reveal new layers of the theme to emerge. The structure followed the dramaturgy of a ritual that represents a key element in the training and practice of the Sesame Approach to dramatherapy, in which I was trained at The Royal Central School of Speech and Drama in London 2005–2007 (Bruun, 2012, Hougham, 2006, Pearson, Smail and Watts, 2013). The main event represents the anti-structure of the ritual where liminality and the space of betwixt-and-between may challenge habitual thinking and feeling responses and in turn, when addressed in the bridge-out, may inspire new patterns to emerge. The bridge-out, in this Jungian-based approach, is essential to wind down and return to the everyday reality because lingering experientially in the embodied imagination during the main event, may provide new insights and transformative learning, individually and collectively. Finally, the here-and-now reality is reinforced making sure that everybody is grounded before the session ends.

After a short warmup in a standing circle tuning in to the workshop together, the group was moving freely in the space sounding together and little by little invited to get into an introspective mode without eye contact. For the bridge-in, the whole group created a sculpt together in silence of a mountain. Then the theme of Echo was introduced with Wordsworth's (2018) poem from 1806. The poem was recited twice and the second time, the group was asked to pick a word or sentence that appealed to them in that moment. Still in the sculpt of the mountain, the group then improvised together starting with one voice at a time repeating their fragment of the poem until everybody was speaking and listening at the same time. The cacophony then continued as a free improvisation as the mountain dissolved and everybody moved freely in the space again ending in a circle to listen to the story of Echo, retold and spoken by me (Bruun, 2016).

The main event was organized around the enactment of the story, prepared in four parts by four groups working in each corner of the workshop space:

1   Echo presented as a talkative and inventive nymph that deceives Juno
2   Juno's discovery of betrayal and the curse of Echo
3   Echo falls in love and is rejected by Narcissus, an active young man hunting with his peers
4   Echo withdraws and her body fades away: 'her bones were transformed into rocks and there was nothing left than her voice' (Bruun, 2016)

The story as rendered by Ovid is also the story of Narcissus, yet for our investigation, Echo was the protagonist, and therefore the ending focussed on her fate and voice. This meant ending the exploration before Narcissus is cursed by Nemesis to fall in love with his own visual reflection. It was equally important to introduce Echo before the curse, as a lively and able speaker, one might even say manipulative and entertaining. The theme of eroticism does not only link to Jupiter's sexual lust, but also to Echo and Narcissus. In Latin, Ovid plays with call and response between the two, in the most ingenious way, as highlighted by Geneviève Lively (2011: 51). When Narcissus hears Echo, he invites her to join him: 'Come here and let us meet [*huc coamus*]', he says. Echo, only able to repeat the last syllables, replies, 'Let us meet [*coamus*]'. This reply, without the *huc*, is naughty and directly alludes to coitus. This moment of misunderstanding between Narcissus and Echo leads to the climax of the story when Echo rushes forward in passion only for Narcissus to reject her. Her love unrequited, she withdraws hurt and her body wastes away.

After about ten minutes of preparation, the whole story was enacted as a continuous sequence. Starting from their corner of the room, each of the four groups took the whole play space in the middle of the room, one after the other while the other groups witnessed the performance. Afterward, to bridge-out, everybody was asked to linger a moment with their experiences of the enactments, as performer and witness and to reflect on their subjective experience of what attracted and repulsed them. The rationale behind this lingering was to allow the experience of the main event to *echo* within. To end the bridge-out, everybody expressed attraction and repulsion in individual sculptures and sounds. The workshop concluded with grounding, returning to the bridge-in exercise the group was asked to recreate the shape of the mountain, with the same or different shapes than during the bridge-in. Together and with help of a cymbal, there was the build-up to a vocal climax when the mountain split, and everybody came to rest in nature as individual rocks. To end the workshop, Wright taught the group a folk song from his younger days, 'I wish I was a rock sitting on a hill' (Adams, no date). The rocks were brought to life and the session ended in playful movement and sound.

## Reflections

The Echo workshop integrated dramatherapy and voicework practice. The purpose was to allow for somatic resonances of any kind to connect to imaginative spaces within and without, subjectively and intersubjectively. We wanted Echo to remind us of our uniqueness and our connectedness. Breath and voice touches on this in a very direct and physical way – and in present time. This aligns with Pitruzzella (2018) who elaborates on how intersubjectivity is part of our nature and foundation for our relational capacity. Another pioneer of dramatherapy, Roger Grainger (1934–2015) interestingly refers directly to Echo in his writings on imagination as the space that 'sets me free to pursue the completeness I long for and do not find anywhere except in encountering the otherness which establishes my own very separate personal identity' (Duggan and Grainger, 1997: 18). By this, he points to the 'disturbance' Echo represents, the immediate resonance within us, that which is different from me and therefore, as Grainger explains, 'establishes my own very separate identity' (Duggan and Grainger, 1997: 18). He continues, '[t]his is a doctrine of imagination which allows it to perform a completely different role from that of an expression of the self (like Echo's distorted expression deconstructs meaning) – *that of moving beyond itself to find a new way of being itself* [my emphasis]' (Duggan and Grainger, 1997: 18). As I understand it, Grainger aligns himself with Bachelard in acknowledging the autonomy of the poetic image and the liberation it may represent from rigid patterns, be it of thought or action.

These are the teachings of Echo reminding us of a deep knowing within that connects us to ourselves and other living beings. The resonance of Echo, as immediate acoustic response, likens the pre-linguistic and playful communication between infant and carer and, as I have demonstrated with the workshop, Echo and echoing invites an embodied awareness of immediate pre-linguistic responding in play that underpins the imaginative space as relational and sensory. For Bachelard (2014: 28) this is the protected place of daydreaming and the emphasis on daydreaming as a healthy driving force cannot be stressed enough. Bachelard introduces the image of the house to hold this inner experience for the mind to wander intuitively between past, present and future. Although his notion of the house as a child's safe spot may seem outdated, Bachelard's point is still relevant concerning our need to feel safe in our bodies and experience containment when the mind wanders and needs space to integrate thoughts, memories and dreams. To this, Bachelard states that '[t]he binding principle in this integration is the daydream' (Bachelard, 2014: 28). This has little to do with house in a literal or nostalgic sense, rather it is the place within us where our embodied intention for healthy self-regulation dwells. This is engrained in our biology (Cavalli and Heard, 2019) and by that, encompassing our subjective bodies connecting us across time and space. This is relevant for all relationships, including for therapy, in the same way as the notion of *Poiesis* and its healing power that in reality is the restauration of the imagination, as asserted by Levine (1997: 42). It is worth noting that Berry understands Echo as a therapist's capacity for inner listening, resonating with the fundamentals of dramatherapy of balancing under- and over-distance (Landy, 1994). She writes that '[t]he point is not distance between analyst and analysand, but intra-psychic distance, distance *within* the psyche' (Berry, 1982: 123).

Bachelard often comes back to Rilke who said that '[t]hrough every human being, unique space, intimate space, opens up to the world ...' (Bachelard, 2014: 218). For Bachelard, there exists the coexistence of images of intimacy and distance, '[f]or each object, distance is the present, the horizon exists as much as the center' (Bachelard, 2014: 219). This entails, as I understand it, that we can experience this coexistence, as coexisting *reality*, rather than as a tension of two opposites. This space is empty *and* full, 'the space of intimacy and world space – blend' (Bachelard, 2014: 219). Bachelard continues, '[w]hen human solitude deepens, then the two immensities touch and become identical', and in this space we are present with 'countless presences', never alone (Bachelard, 2014: 219). Bachelard invites us to enter this space where intimacy and vastness blend. In theory, this was also the space we wanted to frame during the Echo workshop that would allow for each participant to connect to their own subjective poetic experience. This agrees with dramatherapy that aims to develop reflexive imagination that stays connected with realities without and within, such as argued by Pitruzzella (2018). This is in line with Bachelard (2014: 218) who explains that 'to give an object poetic space is to give it more space than it has objectivity; or, better still, it is following the expansion of its intimate space'.

What I intend to stress here is that when we, as living beings, are shaped *by* the world, this does not only refer to the world without, but also to the world *within,* which is the space where we are surrounded by 'countless presences' (Rilke in Bachelard, 2014: 219). Echo's space is full and empty at the same time, and by that, it resonates with Bachelard's poetic imagination. The resonance from Echo is in the present, like poetic images, surprising and coming from seemingly nowhere, yet corresponding deep within our being. Echo's acoustic mirroring distorts and deconstructs meaning, as a regression to speech before language and as sound only. When we can listen in this space – we may not only discover the immediate pleasures of daydreaming and poetry, but we may also land in the shared intersubjective space where we are safe and protected, not as in a lost paradise or in a fantasy, but as in a felt and embodied self-contained reality. This is where we gain courage and inspiration to change our thinking and understand ourselves and others as performative beings, told and retold, again and again, trusting and listening to our ability for *Poiesis*.

## References

Adams, D. (no date) *Well, I Wish I was a Rock*. Available at: https://www.youtube.com/watch?v=B0iYBgr9Wsc

Bachelard, G. and Gaudin, C. (1987) *On Poetic Imagination and Reverie*. Rev. edn. Dallas, Tex: Spring Publications.

Bachelard, G. (2014) *The Poetics of Space*. Penguin Classics.

Baker, F. and Uhlig, S. (2011) *Voicework in Music Therapy: Research and Practice*. Jessica Kingsley Publishers.

Balzac, H. d. (1845) *The Unknown Masterpiece*. https://www.gutenberg.org/ebooks/23060

Berry, P. (1982) *Echo's Subtle Body: Contributions to an Archetypal Psychology*. Spring Publications.

Bruun, E. (2015) 'Listen carefully', *Dramatherapy*, 37(1), pp. 3–14.

Bruun, E.F. (1981) *Le chef-d'oeuvre inconnu inconnu - une lecture critique de Le Chef-d'oeuvre inconnu de Honoré de Balzac*, MPhil Dissertation, Norway: University of Oslo.

Bruun, E.F. (2012) 'Dramatherapy with homeless clients: The necessary theatre', *Dramatherapy*, 34(3), pp. 139–149.

Bruun, E.F. and Wright, D.K. (2013) 'Drama, Heart and Soul: Understanding the Relationship Between the Unique Inner Voice, Heart Intelligence and the Intelligence of Feeling', in Pitruzzella, S., Ross, M. and Scoble, S. (ed.) *Arts Therapies and The Intelligence of Feeling*. Plymouth: University of Plymouth Press, pp. 61–71.

Bruun, E.F. (2016) The Story of Echo retold.

Bruun, E.F. (2021) 'In Front of Me: Fitzmaurice Voicework® as Transformative Practice', in Kapadocha, C. (ed.) *Somatic Voices in Performance and Beyond*. London: Routledge Voices Studies Series.

Cavalli, G. and Heard, E. (2019) 'Advances in epigenetics link genetics to the environment and disease', *Nature*, 571(7766), pp. 489–499. doi: 10.1038/s41586-019-1411-0

Cavarero, A. (2005) *For More Than One Voice: Toward a Philosophy of Vocal Expression*. Stanford, Calif: Stanford University Press.

*Centre Artistique Internationale Roy Hart*. Available at: https://roy-hart-theatre.com/ (Accessed: 11.07.2021 2021).

Duggan, M. and Grainger, R. (1997) *Imagination, Identification and Catharsis in Theatre and Therapy*. Jessica Kingsley Publishers.

*European Federation of Dramatherapy*. Available at: https://www.efdramatherapy. com/conference-2016-romania (Accessed: 12.07.2021 2021).

Fitzmaurice, C. (2015) 'Breathing matters', *Voice and Speech Review*, 9(1), pp. 61–70. doi: 10.1080/23268263.2015.1014191

Hougham, R. (2006) 'Numinosity, symbol and ritual in the Sesame approach', *Dramatherapy*, 28(2), pp. 3–7.

Jennings, S. (1994) *The Handbook of Dramatherapy*. London: Routledge.

Knill, P.J., Levine, E.G. and Levine, S.K. (2005) *Principles and Practice of Expressive Arts Therapy: Towards a Therapeutic Aesthetics*. Jessica Kingsley Publishers.

Landy, R.J. (1994) *Drama Therapy: Concepts, Theories, and Practices*. Springfield, Ill: Charles C Thomas.

Langley, D.M. (2006) *An Introduction to Dramatherapy*. United Kingdom: Sage Publications Ltd.

Levine, S.K. (1997) *Poiesis: The Language of Psychology and the Speech of the Soul*. London: J. Kingsley Publ.

Levine, S.K. (2009) *Trauma, Tragedy, Therapy: The Arts and Human Suffering*. Jessica Kingsley. Available at: http://search.ebscohost.com/login.aspx?direct=true&db= nlebk&AN=299393&site=ehost-live

Liveley, G. (2011) *Ovid's 'Metamorphoses': A Reader's Guide*. London: London: Bloomsbury Publishing Plc.

Low, D. (1992) 'Merleau-Ponty's Intertwined Notions of Subjectivity and Inter-subjectivity', *International Studies in Philosophy*, 24, pp. 45–64.

Merleau-Ponty, M. (2012) *Phenomenology of Perception*. Florence, United Kingdom: Taylor & Francis Group.

Pearson, J., Smail, M. and Watts, P. (2013) *Dramatherapy with Myth and Fairytale: The Golden Stories of Sesame*. London and Philadelphia: Jessica Kingsley Publishers.

Pikes, N. (2019) *Dark Voices: The Genesis of Roy Hart Theatre*. 3rd edn. Zurich, Switzerland: Pikes.

Pitruzzella, S. (2013) 'Passions, Reason and Imagination in Blake's Myth: A Guide for Arts Therapists', in Pitruzzella, S., Ross, M. and Scoble, S. (eds.) *Arts Therapies and The Intelligence of Feeling*. Plymouth: University Press of Plymouth, pp. 73–87.

Pitruzzella, S. (2018) 'The space that divides and connects.' Betweenness and the intersubjective perspective', *Dramatherapy: The Journal of the Association for Dramatherapists*, 39(1), pp. 3–15. doi: 10.1080/02630672.2018.1432669

Ross, M. (2013) 'Whistling in the Dark: The Intelligence of Feeling Revisited', in Pitruzzella, S., Ross, M. and Scoble, S. (eds.) *Arts Therapies and The Intelligence of Feeling*. Plymouth: University of Plymouth Press, pp. 13–33.

Winnicott, D.W. (1971) *Playing and Reality*. London: Tavistock.

Witkin, R.W. (1974) *The Intelligence of Feeling*. London: Heinemann.

Wordsworth, W. (2018) *Poetical Works of William Wordsworth*. [S.l.]: Seltzer Books.

# 2 How Hut Making in Dramatherapy Created a Therapeutic Play Space

*Angie Richardson*

*My legs stick out awkwardly from under a chair, my adult body contorts to fit into the tiny space I have been allocated to be my bed as I lie alongside the bodies of children who fit snugly and easily into this makeshift home. Chairs and fabrics form the elaborate whare[1] they have proudly built together for 'How Maui slowed the Sun', the Maori myth we are enacting.*

This chapter will explore the journey of hut making which became the focal activity for a group of children participating in weekly dramatherapy sessions at their school in Aotearoa, New Zealand. Our sessions were held in a space that had a multitude of uses, was not private and where we were often interrupted by staff. This questionable therapeutic space was also contained within the uncertain and challenging backdrop of the worldwide Covid pandemic, with a four-week lockdown that interrupted our time together. This chapter presents as a case study with vignettes from sessions that tell the story of the work that unfolded. The discussion that follows seeks to untangle the pertinent threads, including the therapeutic benefits for the children who manipulated, and shape shifted the dramatherapy space we were inhabiting through hut making. I will incorporate Māori terms within the text as an acknowledgement that I am a dramatherapist working in Aotearoa and some of the children in the group identified as Māori and are tangata whenua[2] of this land.

## Introduction

Years of clinical experience working as a dramatherapist with children have embedded certain protocols that I consider necessary to create a therapeutic environment within which to physically work. This came to the fore when I found myself navigating a complicated working space when contracted to deliver therapy in a rural primary school in Te Tai Tokerau.[3] Funding had been granted to the school from the Ministry of Education to support and resource tamariki,[4] who may have experienced heightened adverse effects from Covid lockdowns. Teachers nominated students who

DOI: 10.4324/9781003252399-4

presented with a range of whanau[5] related issues and life difficulties which had given rise to behavioural and emotional concerns. I first met with them individually administering an arts-based assessment to ascertain an appropriate fit for either individual creative arts therapy or to participate in a dramatherapy group. Those in the dramatherapy group who consistently attended school and therefore most of the group sessions, ranged in age from seven to ten years and included boys and girls.

The school had burgeoning enrolments and additional classrooms were delayed due to Covid lockdowns, so space was a scarce commodity. I was given the use of the school's multi-purpose room for the dramatherapy sessions. While a good size and positioned to one side of the school, it had the effect of feeling somewhat like a fishbowl with large glass windows and sliding doors. The inner wall was also glass and through this was the school library which was having to be used as a classroom for the new entrant children. It fulfilled its multi-purpose title accommodating many different activities within the school and also doubled up as the staff room. This was to become problematic as many people needed access to it even though I had been assured it was booked exclusively for my group on the allocated day.

Initial therapeutic aims promoted developing a nurturing therapeutic alliance to enable the children to feel safe along with building group cohesion through co-operative dramatic play. Other projected outcomes included growing self-esteem through being witnessed and fostering the ability to feel confident to contribute creative ideas. These sat alongside individual goals for personal or social needs such as developing positive relationships with peers. I was acutely aware of the importance of building a strong foundation at the beginning of the work, one which implicated the space we were to inhabit. According to Case and Dalley

> The space is essentially a private place with a firm outer boundary which enables a sense of containment, security, freedom from intrusion and an atmosphere of calm and reflection. The layout, organisation and design of the room becomes a creative 'arena' or potential space for setting up and maintaining the ongoing therapeutic encounter between therapist, client and art materials
>
> (Case and Dalley, 2014: 60)

As the therapeutic modality was dramatherapy, I provided props and materials required for the session and to furnish the scenes of stories but my initial understanding was that the space would at least meet my expectation as detailed by Case and Dalley of being private and free from interruptions. That this turned out not to be the case gave rise to some interesting reflections and adjustments as I grappled with what it means to be a flexible practitioner in a way I had not experienced before.

**Vignette 1**

The morning of the first session arrived and I pushed the staff dining tables to one side and set up chairs in a circle, which only slightly encroached into the kitchen facilities. Five of the seven tamariki were eventually corralled from their classrooms and together we expectantly, albeit hesitantly, sat in our circle to meet and greet each other. However, we were not alone. There were a couple of lingering staff members who seemed quite comfortable to remain where they were, drinking their coffee and chatting. I explained that our session was about to start and became somewhat troubled when they didn't seem to comprehend the significance of this. I then felt compelled to offer a firm invitation for them to move on so I could attend to the children who were now wriggling about in their chairs with nervous impatience.

The sessions followed a three-phase process of warm-up, the developmental phase and then closure, described by Cattanach as being the 'structure [that] is needed to help the group function in the language of dramatic action, to hold the group together and to create a mood and environment which can stimulate creative work' (Cattanach, 1993a: 37). While the physical environment provides the physical boundary for this to happen within, it is also useful to have clear guidelines to frame up how the work is to be done. This supports the therapist's holding of the group and supports members on how to be a member of this particular group. Our initial warmup started with the negotiation and creation of a group treaty for how we were to work together. It was helpful to refer to this when the children were navigating their way with each other, particularly for one young participant who struggled to '*be with*' and remain in active relationship with the rest of the group. While it was useful to manage relational connecting, I had not foreseen that a discussion around how to treat the teacher's furniture would also have been constructive!

The boundaries of both the space and our relationship were tested early on when warmup exercises included moving around the room. The seemingly innocuous couches and coffee tables became a highly enticing playground for the children to climb over and hide under. I imagine the fact that this area of the room was usually off limits to the children, being the teacher's refuge at break times, leading it to becoming a magnet for vigorous and excited exploration. Despite the room having the immediate and desired result of engendering a shared playful energy into the group, the somewhat questionable motivation and direction of this play had me feeling somewhat panicky. Firstly, about any resulting damage to said furniture and secondly about a teacher popping in and bearing witness to this somewhat out of control action. Although it had not been explicitly addressed during our treaty discussion, there was undoubtably an unspoken understanding that this behaviour would not be allowed under 'usual school circumstances' and there was an obvious reluctance to stop. I also noted how quickly shyness and hesitation can dissipate in the spirit of such conspiratorial play.

With somewhat stern encouragement the group reassembled in the chair circle, which became the constant anchor to return to when things felt too unwieldly and when form was dissipating. In the developmental phase of the first session, I introduced the story, 'Where the Wild Things are' by Maurice Sendak (1963) for the children to enact. In retrospect, there was certainly an irony in this, but my initial choice to use this text was rooted in role play, and it was a story I had effectively used many times with both children and adults. It provides delightful scope for some simple improvisation that can encourage those not versed in acting to have a go at theatrical expression. There was a sense of uncertain apprehension in the group as I invited them to take on roles and enact the opening scene with Max and his mother.

I had aspirations of tamariki taking on the dramatic representation of being the walls of Max's bedroom transforming into a forest as 'his ceiling hung with vines and the walls became the world all around' (Sendak, 1963). However, this became a free for all as they dropped their allocated roles in favour of becoming the Wild Things, demonstrating a wondrous capacity to play to the beat of their own drum rather than a more gently facilitated and contained enactment led by me and my drum. It was a bit disconcerting to see how quickly the therapeutic aims of increasing spontaneity and empowerment had been met. The uptake of the monster roles was possibly aided by the odd aesthetics of the costumes I had offered: a range of colourful knotted scarves which formed a dress of sorts that could easily go over their heads. In Jennings' Embodiment-Projection-Role (EPR) model she describes how costumes along with other props support the child in becoming a character that has charge over the play action (2002: 7). This certainly proved to be the case in this situation, and the children were having a great deal of fun. My question was whether this was the result of careful planning or if it had been the somewhat raucous elements of our time together!

At the beginning of our second session, navigating the space was again challenging. We were interrupted once again, this time by a teacher-aide needing to get things from the kitchen and a caretaker who insisted on emptying the dishwasher, even with the 'PLEASE DO NOT ENTER, DRAMATHERAPY IN PROGRESS' sign on the door. The group was eager to re-engage with Sendak's story and so on went the costumes. One young girl proposed that the small innocuous pile of fabrics situated by my props bag could be used to make a house for the story. This one innocent suggestion inadvertently set the scene for how our work together was to flow, albeit more of a tumbling than a smooth sailing.

Immediately there was a sense of purposeful energy as they tackled the challenge of building a 'house'. Chairs were hauled about, and different strategies tried to organize the fabrics into roofs that when placed on the chairs would also serve as walls. What evolved was a number of houses rather than one large one, perhaps reflecting the group's identity at that stage of being a collection of individuals rather than a connected community. When they were satisfied with their handywork the dramatic action resumed, however 'Where the Wild Things Are' somehow melded into 'The Three Little Pigs' with the students each having their own 'hut' and the roles for this became quite fluid. Finally, there was another natural transformation into a story about a neighbourhood and the children were more themselves in this rather than playing an imaginary role.

---

**Vignette 2**

In the third session, the children asked if they could make huts again. I had anticipated this request and ensured I brought a large selection of fabrics from my collection. These included one huge piece of lycra with a brightly patterned universe on it and a large variety of other colourful and textured materials. This time they opted to build one big hut for the group and readily set about working co-operatively, planning how and where the different fabrics would best be utilized to create their 'home'. There was a wonderful sense of cohesion, with a clear focus on intent and absorption in the process and an atmosphere of enjoyment as they created together. They were able to demonstrate determination and resourcefulness when dealing with the fickle nature of using fabrics as their building materials. At its completion, which included the careful arrangement of soft fabric on the ground by one of the youngest group members so it would be 'nice and cosy', most of the tamariki were keen to get into the house and start improvising a story about families.

However, even though the hut looked inviting, and the children were welcoming, there was one young boy who refused to go in and hid under the couch curled up in a ball. I tried to engage him gently and playfully, but he ignored me, so I called to the group that I had found a wee baby bird that needed help. Immediately two of the girls 'flew over' and lay close to him being his parents, which he really seemed to like. Other children joined us and we flew about to find food and fed him and he became a very happy baby bird. The theme of home and family was obviously quite triggering for this young person. By utilizing dramatic invention, the couch in effect became a bird's nest. The group then enabled him to join them through sensitive role play in a way that met his emotional needs in that moment. Cattanach captures this capacity of dramatherapy stating, 'Dramatic play is the way children are able to transform experience through the symbolic form of the fictions they create ... Not only do children "try out" possible futures and "act out" problems of the past, but they engage in problem solving in a deep personal way through the fictional present' (1994: 138).

A few days after this session, I found myself having to self-isolate having driven hastily back up North from Tāmaki Makaurau,[6] where Covid-19 had made an abrupt and inconvenient return. With Auckland shut down and its borders closed, Te Tai Tokerau was essentially cut off from the rest of the country and schools in the region were closed for a month. While I remained in good spirits and was resourced and nourished by being close to a beach, I struggled with being unable to see family and friends, who were across the lockdown border. I was also anxious to resume work and I wondered how the tamariki from my group were faring with yet another Covid lockdown and the resulting stressors that they and their whanau would be under. Fortunately for us, while schools remained closed for a sustained period in Auckland, the epicentre of the Covid outbreak, the rest of the schools in the country reopened including schools up North and after four weeks we returned to the dramatherapy space.

## Vignette 3

There was high excitement from the children to be with each other again and they bounced alongside me to the multipurpose room, very keen to get the session underway. They were thrilled when I produced a bag of puppets having promised prior to lockdown that I would bring some in. We used the puppets for a warmup exercise and then they devised the plan of making a home for themselves and the puppets to live in. Out came the fabrics and when they were confident that the *whare* would withstand some lively family interactions, the storying began. This was initiated by one child, who had remained committed to the original story of 'Where the Wild Things Are' and was keen to maintain her role of being the whaea[7] to Max. She proceeded to order everyone to bed and a boisterous improvised game developed of chasing, catching, hiding, being safe and not being safe with the hut being the pivotal place of the action, alongside leaping around the aforementioned furniture.

There was a great deal of boisterous energy expelled. I could only postulate that the copious expunging of energy was perhaps the result of having been penned up in their homes for the past month. I had less energy to spare, having to work twice as hard to crawl through the child-sized hut in an effort to escape bedtime while trying to catch and keep out of reach of what appeared to be my siblings with my alter ego puppet on my hand. There was no clear storyline, it felt incoherent and loose, more like a dressed-up version of tag with the hut offering a boundary of safety and non-safety as a play theme in the therapeutic space. At this moment it did not feel like there was any frame to this action and the boundaries were blurred.

For two sessions we did not play at making huts, instead, we engaged in different improvisational approaches for the developmental phase of the session. On reflection, I was aware that the children's enthusiasm had dwindled, and the collective energy of the group was disrupted. I realized there was some unfinished business with what we had started. While the act of creating huts may have seemed in the first instance a random activity that could lead to incoherent and wild play, it was in its absence that a true potency was revealed. Thus, we plunged back into the fertile territory of hut making.

**Vignette 4**

I chose to introduce the Maori legend 'How Māui Slowed The Sun' to frame the activity of hut making and the children were inspired to take on the different roles it offered. Māui is a well-known cultural hero in Maori mythology, and he embarks on numerous exploits and adventures to help his people. This story seemed to really ignite the children's imaginations. While tamariki swapped roles from week to week from Māui to the sun to the brothers, they also created new roles such as the moon and the ocean. The fabrics returned and were transformed to support these role developments. A long blue silky fabric became the oceans flowing cloak where the other children would swim on top of while journeying to find the sun. A ritual ensued of opening the story by making the *whare* within which Māui and his whanau would settle into sleep before being awoken by the sun banging a loud gong. As the story developed and evolved, more huts were needed as the sun and the moon decided they needed their own homes.

The storyline was not strictly adhered to, rather it was a springboard for the children to actively engage in ways that they each wanted but also where they contributed to the aesthetics of the whole. The children grew in confidence to expand their role repertoire and were gloriously creative in how they did this, creating their own sense of dramatic style to colour the story. In effect they were acting as if they were performing, they were undeniably themselves but there was a different edge and quality to the dramatic play. They were exploring the play space in more sophisticated ways. It is likely they had transitioned through developmental stages during these sessions. Cattanach believes this is an important task of the dramatherapist, to ensure the facilitation of the developmental flow. She articulates this saying 'This flow should appear seamless as the group move along the developmental continuum in each individual dramatherapy session and through the process as a whole' (1993a: 39).

## Discussion

In exploring the significance of hut making, American educator David Sobel, well known for his seminal work on the philosophy of place-based education, has written widely about the importance of this activity. Sobel researched that making huts, forts and dens are a universal childhood activity that play an important role in children's development across cultures. He writes, 'In these secret places, children develop and control environments of their own and enjoy freedom from the rules of the adult world' (Sobel, 2019:1). One developmental function is that as children begin to have a sense of independence from their parents/caregivers and explore their environment, they desire a separate space. Younger children create such spaces in the home by placing blankets over tables and chairs for example and then from age 7 onwards they seek to make them outside the home (Sobel, 2002: 61). I posit that within the confines of our therapeutic space the children intuitively and organically latched onto the hut making as an integral part of our process as a means to create a haven within an environment that on many levels may have felt chaotic and uncertain.

The therapeutic space was also contained within the uncertain and stress inducing backdrop of the worldwide Covid pandemic including the four-week lockdown that occurred during our time together. Undoubtedly, within the taxing environment of Covid, families were experiencing hardship and uncertainty as an added dimension to cope with. As Carol Stock Kranowitz, a multi arts educator, states, 'Forts help children reset their stressed bodies and brains', (Kranowitz cited in Margolin, 2020: 20). Huts allow children to inhabit a space that they can call home, where they have authority around how they are built and what happens in them. Some of the tamariki in the group had or still were experiencing a multiplicity of challenges in the home environment, such as poverty, whanau separation, dislocation and loss. Their sense of having any control or sense of agency over different aspects of their lives was likely very low which may have been one of the underlying motivators for the fascination the children showed for repeatedly engaging in this activity. Here they could create a safe and stable home that did not house family stress or tension or conflict that may have been present in some whanau homes.

It may also have underscored the elongated timeframe to which they dedicated themselves to hut building each session. I had always been curious about the amount of time engaged in the creation of the huts as opposed to the amount of time that was then left for some dramatic play to entail within them. While I eventually came to see the benefit of the hut making process, for some time I felt the need to expediate this and get into the drama, the 'acting' element of our sessions that was my experience and training. It was therefore a relief when I read British dramatherapist Amy Willshire extol the virtues of hut making, saying that this is her most used resource going into primary schools and doing dramatherapy with students. She explained how often making the den is the main therapeutic activity, where the children take the time to make a space with fabrics that is just for them or others they may be working with (Willshire, 2019).

Along with the creation of the huts, another standout feature of our work was the dominant theme of family that emerged strongly through the children's own devised play and became the focus of story enactments. This theme which developed so quickly seemed to serve two purposes. Firstly, it underscored the significance of whanau/family in relation to their own lives and secondly it became a means of the group bonding quickly. What we enacted we also became. The individuals in the group were concerned for each other and it became a group that felt very comfortable in being together, like a good-enough family. This was demonstrated in their capacity to be with each other in a robust and exploratory way. For some participants, one function of the dramatherapy group was to develop more positive relationships with their peers. Madan (2010) suggests that dramatic play is a safe way to work through difficult experiences and impeded developmental stages which can facilitate emotional and interpersonal learning. She writes, 'Especially for a child whose attachment processes have been disrupted … play can have an important role in helping facilitate attachments in a non-intrusive, mutually negotiated way' (Madan, 2010: 266).

The huts and the interactions they invoked through the theme of families became the container that could safely host this multi-layered relational exploration. As noted previously, one participant was very keen to play the role of Mother whenever she could, enjoying the chance to boss and nurture 'her' children. This was also demonstrated in the example where one child became a baby bird and the others' 'mothered' it. Another paradoxical and poignant moment was another instance where we had a group member purposefully destroying another child's hut as they deliberately walked through it. The owner occupier of the hut was distraught by this desecration especially when the other child refused to apologize. It seemed the distress was twofold: the sanctity of the hut was violated and pulled down along with the trust in their relationship. This rupture was eventually able to be repaired after a deliberate intervention on my part to secure reparation through dramatic intervention.

While it is important to tease apart the different strands that making huts played in creating a space that enabled therapeutic work to take place so too must I consider my own part in this process. As indicated at the beginning of this chapter, most of the tamariki in this group had/were experiencing a range of difficult circumstances or familial situations. Underlying this is the cultural milieu we each carried and for some of these tamariki so too was unconscious material arising from systemic inequalities and intergenerational trauma brought about by Pākehā[8] colonization. The students in the group identified as being either Pākehā and/or Maori and I identify as Pākehā. Another dimension was that I was not from Te Tai Tokerau, I was new to the area, I did not have a prior relationship to the school, the community or the land. I was going through my own process of what it meant to be living in a rural context and what lens I carried in relation to this.

In effect this space was the children's place however I was the one welcoming them into it, providing the conditions within which they could safely explore their monsters. We come with our own realities that hold our ideas of identity and place which are culturally constructed. These aspects of self come into play in the therapeutic space. Jackson challenges therapists to have 'cultural humility' to consider cultural variables in our work with different client groups and to question how to be with this (2021:76). I surmise that the hut building became the physical and symbolic threshold for our liminal meeting. Here the children had agency and a level of control, creating an even playing field where we could meet on equal relational terms. Inside the huts 'playing' at families they were able to invite me into the space and into relationship with them as opposed to me making the invitations. We were able to co-create authentic experiences that were meaningful, that valued the difference each of us brought (Malchiodi, 2020: 57). As this evolved, we were indeed companioning each other, we were kindred spirits, able to more fully surrender to the unconscious play material that was needed by the children. (Powis, 2010: 232).

What also became strikingly apparent was that these children were in need of play, an adult to play 'with' and also to be 'seen' by. For those children affected by trauma and disrupted attachment, neurobiology is helping us better understand how this can impact their physiological development. It can have the effect of interfering with a natural ability to be playful and creative (Malchiodi, 2020: 33–32). Chaotic and/or stressed family lives, busy classrooms, modern devices that children spend time on rather than physical play, these factors -among others- contribute to an issue that I would label as 'play deprivation'. The developmental stage that occupied the children for so long around the physical making of the hut, the arranging of the inside, the 'childlike' feel to this indicated the children were in need of some reparative play. Here was an opportunity to engage meaningfully and deeply in what it means to be playful, to have an experience of exploring the environment in a fun way and to be supported and held as it were while doing it.

Cattanach speaks to the healing such spaces as huts and dens can provide being the borderlands of children's social worlds. She cites the work of Winnicott (1971) who recognizes the importance of the relationship between therapist and child client while playing here and sees the psychic space between the two as being like the potential space between child and mother (1994: 137). One of my roles as the therapist was to be the 'good enough' mother who can be relied on to set up the play, provide the materials needed as well as play with them. For the story of Māui, I would hide sticks prior to the session beginning and the children would find and gather them to make a 'fire' to cook the fish they caught. Such a simple activity and yet each time the children were so delighted to hunt them out and bring them back to show me.

Perhaps for this reason, the ending of our time together was particularly hard. The contract came to its conclusion near the close of the school year and as I was preparing to relocate back to Tāmaki Makaurau over the Summer holidays, there was not the possibility of seeing if we could extend the programme. Many tears were shed, and hugs were had as we farewelled and thanked each other for our time together. That multipurpose room had seen much aroha[9] and magic being shared in that play space and it was heart-rending to say goodbye. This piece of work was a privilege to be part of and I am in gratitude to the tamariki I was fortunate to work with, it has shifted something within. I continue to grow and evolve as a therapist. Taku mihi aroha ki a koutou tamariki mā, mō ngā mahi katoa kua oti i a tātau. Thank you, children, my heartfelt thanks to you, for all the work we have done.

## Conclusion

While to all intents and purposes the therapeutic space the dramatherapy group inhabited was less than ideal, we were able to adapt and make it a safe and robust working space. The hut making ritual which was a key feature of our therapeutic work in turn also helped to establish a space for a dramatic reality to be entered into, inviting potent play to emerge. In this regard, I am able to concur with Grainger (cited in Jennings, 1994: 7), who has found that sometimes the most 'unsuitable' dramatherapeutic room has produced the most significant experiences. I agree with the observation Jones makes that as dramatherapists we respond and work with the situations our clients bring, therefore the practice of dramatherapy 'varies enormously' (2014: 10). Then I would add, occasionally our practice is provoked and shaken up due to the unique nature of a client/group, place and time as happened to me here. This experience has gifted me an appreciation of how to approach and *be with the therapeutic space* in a very different way.

Hut making captured the children's imagination and propelled the theme of 'families' into the spotlight. I bore witness that the children wanted to repeat and 'indulge' in the creation process which they themselves had initiated and which organically manifested as the central work in our time together. Initially, as our cultural worlds converged and collided in the ecotone of our coming together, there seemed to be a clumsiness to what was unfolding. There was no flow no ease. In reflection, I kept coming back to blaming the space, acknowledging my own discomfort and I assumed the children might be feeling the same. But there were many more layers than the inconvenience of someone wandering through the room to make a coffee. When I was able to let go of my 'cultural' assumption of what constitutes therapy and dramatic play and become the guest to their hosting and knowing, then there was juice, then there was flow, then we were in the groove.

Hut making also supported the development of 'creative courage' in the children, where they could use and develop their imaginations to assist them to discover how to be more fully themselves and how to be with the challenges of life (Malchiodi, 2020: 35). Play itself becomes the space that houses that development, as Anderson-Warren and Grainger explain it, 'For the child ... play is workshop, laboratory, studio – the place and time for imagination to forge a creative response to life' (2000: 53). This work has taken me to a place where the issue of 'play deprivation' has become paramount. Whanau trauma, social and cultural dislocation, intergenerational and systemic inequality can result in chaotic lives for families that impact their capacity to provide rich, nourishing and play-full childhood environments. Likewise, there are numerous life stressors including current ones related to the covid pandemic, that affect all families and have a bearing on how children are played with.

Dramatherapy is an approach that naturally lends itself to children having an opportunity to engage in dramatic interventions where they can do the developmental play-work they need to do. This case study has demonstrated how utilizing hut making in dramatherapy is a process that can support this type of therapeutic approach. Here also the children's capacity to play expanded as their repertoire of dramatic expression grew through accessing their innate imaginations and unique creativity. As Sobel so aptly states, 'If we allow children to shape their own small worlds in childhood, then they will grow up knowing and feeling that they can participate in shaping the big world tomorrow'. (1993,161).

Ma te huru huru, Ka rere te manu

Adorn the bird with feathers so it can soar[10]

## Notes

1  'Whare' is the Māori word for hut/house
2  'tangata whenua' Māori are the tangata whenua (indigenous people) of Aotearoa New Zealand
3  'Te Tai Tokerau' is the Māori term for Northland, Aotearoa
4  'tamariki' is the Māori word for children
5  'whanau' is the Māori word for family
6  'Tāmaki Makaurau' is the Māori name for Auckland
7  'whaea' is the Māori term for mother
8  'Pākehā' is the Māori word for New Zealander of European descent
9  'Aroha' is the Māori word for love and affection
10  A Māori Whakataukī /proverb

## Bibliography

Anderson-Warren, M. and Grainger, R. (2000) *Practical Approaches to Dramatherapy The Shield of Perseus*. London: Jessica Kingsley Publishers.

Case, C. and Dalley, T. (2014) *The Handbook of Art Therapy*. 3rd Edition. Hove, East Sussex: Routledge.

Cattanach, A. (1993a) 'The developmental model of dramatherapy', in Jennings, S., Cattanach, A., Mitchell, S., Chesner, A. & Meldrum, B. (eds.) *The Handbook of Dramatherapy*. London: Routledge, pp. 28–40.

Jackson, L.C. (2021) *Cultural Humility in Art Therapy: Applications for Practice, Research, Social Justice, Self Care and Pedagogy*. London: Jessica Kingsley Publishers.

Jennings, S. (1994). 'Prologue' in Jennings, S., Cattanach, A., Mitchell, S., Chesner, A. & Meldrum, B. (eds.) *The Handbook of Dramatherapy*. London: Routledge, pp. 1–11.

Jennings, S. (2002) *Embodiment-projection-role (EPR)*. [Online] Available at: http://www.suejennings.com/epr.html [Accessed 25 February. 2022].

Jones, P. (2014) 'Opening play: research into play and dramatherapy', in Brock, A., Jarvis, P. & Olusoga, Y. (eds.) *Perspectives on Play: Learning for Life*. 2nd Edition. Oxon: Routledge, pp. 248–268.

Madan, A. (2010) 'Saisir les etoiles: fostering a sense of belonging with child survivors of war', in Jones, P. (ed.). *Drama as Therapy Clinical Work and Research into Practice Volume 2*. East Sussex: Routledge, pp. 260–277.

Malchiodi, C.A. (2020) *Trauma and Expressive Arts Therapy: Brain, Body and Imagination in the Healing Process*. New York: The Guilford Press.

Margolin, S.C. (2020). *Why kids love building forts and why experts say they might need them more than ever*. [Online] Available at: https://www.washingtonpost.com/lifestyle/2020/05/18/why-kids-love-building-forts-why-experts-say-they-might-need-them-more-than-ever/ [Accessed 25 November. 2021]

Powis, C. (2010) 'Cinderella: the role fights back', in Jones, P. (ed.). *Drama as Therapy Clinical Work and Research into Practice Volume 2*. East Sussex: Routledge, pp. 224–246.

Sendak, M. (1963) *Where The Wild Things Are*. London: Random House Children's Publishers.

Sobel, D. (1993/2002). *Children's Special Places: Exploring the Role of Forts, Dens, and Bush Houses in Middle Childhood*. Detroit: Wayne State University Press.

Sobel, D. (2019). *About children's special places*. [Online] Available at: https://www.davidsobelauthor.com/childrens-special-places

Winnicott, D. W. (1971). *Playing and Reality.* Penguin.

Willshire, A. (2019). *The den. A safe space. A space for me. Building. Entering. Inhabiting. Reflecting*. [Online] Available at: https://play-it-through.co.uk/2019/05/30/dens/ [Accessed 13 February 2022]

# 3 Space Plays a Leading Role

## The Therapeutic Power of the Built Environment and Co-Design in Dramatherapy

*Eliza Sweeney*

This chapter presents my initial and ongoing reflections on the power of the external environment to contribute to the therapeutic process in dramatherapy. Supported by theories of environmental psychology it aims to shed light upon the power of the places and the objects within which we work and highlights how a co-design process with clients can be therapeutic. Environmental psychologist Howard Proshansky aptly remarked that 'surprisingly it did not occur to psychologists that perhaps part of the variation involving (psychological) phenomena could be attributed to the nature, meaning, design, organization and use of physical space' (Proshansky, 1976: 205). Before the birth of environmental psychology, since space was never considered to be part of the patient's original problem or pathology, it was never considered to be a potential part of the solution either and I argue that in a therapeutic setting, *where* things happen is critical to knowing *how* and *why* they happen (Warf and Arias, 2014). When I think to the places I have worked, *where* sessions have occurred and *how* the room was designed and arranged has greatly impacted *how* therapy occurs and the quality of that therapy. For the purposes of this chapter, space is viewed as a noun, that three-dimensional space in which objects and people are located such as the buildings, institutions and rooms within which we practice and, inspired by Marcus Doel's suggestion that 'it would be better to approach space as a verb rather than as a noun. *To space* – that's all' (Crang and Thrift, 2000, p. 125), I propose that it is possible to take the gerund form, 'spacing', and bring this into the dramatherapy room. That is to say, that to do dramatherapy, or any art therapy form, is to be in a permanent state of *spacing*. That is to say that in dramatherapy we, the client and the therapist, are in a constant state of discovering, imagining, creating, transforming, shifting and sharing space, both imaginary, emotional, relational and concrete. For the purposes of this chapter, I will be focussing on concrete spaces and their interiors, as they are designed and arranged. It is not my intention to provide a map or manual for how dramatherapy environments should be, as I believe the design of space should remain flexible and responsive to the clients we meet, but rather my intention for this chapter is to open a discussion on some of the effects of the environment, citing a few case studies from my clinical practice as exemplars where the room,

DOI: 10.4324/9781003252399-5

the objects, the design and the arrangement of space become the primary focus and play a leading role. Reflection and analysis are viewed through the lens of psychoanalysis.

Psychiatrist and psychotherapist Michael Fordham (1978) argued that 'just as the analyst needs to be aware of his inner world, so does he need to be aware of parts of himself outside him in the room'(Lingiardi and De Bei, 2011: 390). From Fordham's provocation, I propose that just as the drama therapist must be attuned to the interior worlds of the client and themselves in dramatherapy sessions they must also be conscious and attuned to the exterior universes created and their effect. Over the course of a career as a designer and then drama therapist, I find myself in constant contemplation of the power of the built environment to affect and its potential to be therapeutic. Therapeutic is understood here as any practice, process or product that is relational, inclusive, sensorial, affective, caring and responsible. As a designer, my awareness of space's capacity to alter the meaning of things was limited to the task of creating functional and aesthetic spaces. Shifting my role to drama therapist led me to discovering new meanings about space and place, the effects and *affects* of design, spatial arrangement and how space is relational. For the purposes of this chapter, *affects of design* denotes any design feature that causes affect, emotion, or a coming to consciousness of previously unconscious thought, memory or feeling. I entered the field of dramatherapy viewing the space through the lens of a designer which drew my attention to the signification of the location, the buildings, the interior design and the scenography which housed the dramatherapy sessions, as well as the arrangement and quality of these spaces within which I was training and working. Initially, I would consider the aesthetic qualities of the session environment and their locality – whether we were housed in a public or private institution and the social, political and cultural stakes of this institution, as well as considerations about whether was the room accessible, conducive or restrictive to creativity, comfortable, pleasing, etc. Little by little I began to notice how significantly the space, its context, design and qualities not only impacted the context of the therapy but it was implicit and involved and even sometimes guided the therapy in the process. It became clear to me that the built environment housing any therapeutic session holds an immense capacity to alter the therapeutic process and the ways in which we engage with or ignore the space can have repercussions on our therapeutic practices. I developed an insatiable curiosity to understand the impact of the environment on the therapeutic process. An instinct that reared its head in 2014 during my master's degree upon observing children's interactions with the space in paediatric psychiatry has developed into a part of my professional identity and I maintain my fervent belief and faith in the power of the environment to shape, transform, change and intervene in the therapeutic process across the many forms of art therapy, including dramatherapy. This belief has since been phenomenologically observed and qualitatively documented in my practice and has led to my current doctoral research in architecture that seeks to understand co-design practices as art therapeutic medium.

What follows is the presentation of a few moments over my career where encounters with space and place-making contributed to the therapeutic process in dramatherapy which highlights space as part of the therapeutic solution. The first example details a dramatherapy group in an educational setting where co-design methodologies were implemented in support of the group's need to have their own place in order to work through relational and behavioural challenges. The second example presents a culmination of observations of the child-to-curtain therapeutic relationship in paediatric psychiatry and private practice across a five-year span in the invented '*Julie*', where focus is placed on the central role and use of the curtain object in dramatherapy space

---

**Vignette One**

This first vignette comes from my early work in an educational setting with children from precarious living situations who presented with behavioural, concentration and relational challenges in the school space. The group was made up of 6 10-year-old children. This vignette will attempt to demonstrate how the location of the session affected the children's capacity to engage in the work and how a co-design methodology contributed to healing and transformation. For this group, we were provided with a standard Parisian primary classroom filled with rows of tables and chairs filling the space. In preparation for the sessions, I would arrive early and push back the tables and chairs in order to clear the space in the centre of the classroom. Clearing the space for the children also cleared my mental space, preparing me to welcome and receive their stories, emotions and processes as their therapist. However, while I had the best intentions of preparing the room as such and while the children were thrilled to see their classroom space altered in such a fun way, it seemed to encourage liberal yelling, shouting and exuberant movement and it discouraged focus and involvement the dramatherapy tools I had originally planned. In 1968 Roger Barker, father of ecological (environmental) psychology, put forward his notion of the 'Behaviour Setting' where he emphasized the interdependence between behaviour and the environment. Barker noted that a room furnished with tables and chairs in neat linear rows makes particular demands on the body and behaviour compared to an open learning space that encourages children to run and play (Barker, 1968: 69). He demonstrated how the layout of pedagogical spaces impacts learning, explaining how each type of behaviour is inextricably linked to a particular structure of space. In an educational setting, the classroom is the site of learning and development and this place demands a certain behaviour from its students. Similarly, psychologist Robert Sommer, recognized the phenomena of 'socio-fuge spaces', and subsequently studied the relationship between furniture and conversation in educational spaces, where the orientation of space would have an impact on relationships. Robert Sommer and Helge Olsen (1980) re-designed a college classroom, changing it into a 'soft classroom' that had cushion-covered bench seating, adjustable lighting, a small carpet and some mobiles. This layout and design, compared to traditional classroom settings with rigid table seating arrangements for example, led to an increase in student participation, with the percentage of students speaking up in class almost doubling. A logbook was kept in the classroom and students wrote many positive responses to the new classroom arrangement, and according to Wong, Sommer, & Cook (1992) the room continued to produce an increase in student participation for the following 17 years. It was thus clear that changing the overall design of a learning space can positively affect learning

After a few weeks of juggling the children's desire to run around and my need to get down to business, it occurred to me that the space was communicating the wrong message. Primary children, especially in France, are schooled in rules and regulations from day one. The rules of the traditional classroom were therefore deeply embedded in the group: tables and chairs signified concentration, focus and work and an open space signified free and unstructured play. The classroom space, therefore, dictated much of their behaviour, as Sommer and Olsen have proven decades earlier (1980), and the open space that I had created with the intention to make a 'drama therapeutic space' had not achieved its objective at all. It was clear to me that working in their classroom was not conducive to supporting the therapeutic work and so in discussion with the school Director, we shifted the therapy group to an unused basement space. While a basement evokes images of something sinister, dark and dank, thankfully the room was light-filled and airy with a rounded ceiling that evoked a sense of the mysterious and images of Ali Baba's secret cave. Engaging in a co-design methodology, that promotes collaboration, participation and end-user engagement, the students made decisions about how the space would be redesigned and arranged. They cleared the excess junk (symbolically and literally 'clearing, claiming and sanctifying the space', as Grainger would say (2003)), added a long black cotton curtain to divide the play space from the backstage or 'real life' space, implemented softer lighting with lamps and torches as spotlights strapped to music stands and the students added a colourfully decorated *Please, Do Not Enter* sign on the door during our sessions. Fortunately, we were able to leave the room as we wanted it to be because it was not used for any other purpose other than our group, which I acknowledge was very luxurious indeed. Rather than continuing on with improvisation, role play and other classic dramatherapy exercises, I attuned in to the healing process that occurred in the co-design phase of making our therapeutic space and felt intuitively that continuing with a scenography, architecture and design methodology would respond well to the needs of this group. Over a period of nine months, we went on to building huts and forts out of recycled cardboard, fabric and furniture that became settings within which individual and collective storytelling took place and in a second phase of work, we engaged in a re-design methodology of their home spaces, with a specific focus on their bedrooms. The children would spend time reflecting on their bedroom spaces, often shared with one or more siblings or family members, then they would draw these spaces and imagine how they could re-design a small zone of that room to be entirely their own. One group member slept in a bunk bed with his older sister, he had the lower bunk. So he decided to make a collage of fabric, like a roughly hewn quilt, that he then hung across the whole side of the bunk bed. This created a zone of protection and a place to retreat from the hectic home life. Another group member spent time painting a series of six A3 paintings that she stuck on the wall of her room, on her side of the space. Images of clouds, gardens, fountains, birds and treehouses adorned these colourful pictures and she expressed how one day she would like to live in a treehouse. After building a fort or a hut from chairs and fabric, one member of the group crawled inside and shouted '*You can't come in. No one can break in or tear this down*', signalling the deep need within them to have a safe place that could not be taken away, broken or torn down around them. For context, this participant was adopted from a violent home as a toddler and knowing this background, I understood in this moment that his fear of being taken away from his adoptive family was very present, and that his maladaptive behaviour at school was symptomatic of his feeling that he had not settled into his place in the school group community either.

According to environmental psychologist Howard Proshansky, it is the physical world of the person in the form of rooms, buildings, streets, houses, hospitals, institutions, ad infinitum that contributes to their development and that the arrangement of furniture in someone's home is a subtle expression of their values. Environmental psychologists invite us to consider how certain concepts such as 'self-esteem', 'self-identity' or 'behaviour' are influenced by the physical environment (Proshansky, Ittelson and Rivlin, 1970). The idea that space contributes to self-building contributes to the conversation on dramatherapy spaces that are, potentially, in constant 'co-construction' (Hocini, Le Run and Potel Baranes, 2006) of selves: the client's self, the therapist's self and the relationship between the two.

The therapeutic effect of the spatial shift from classroom to basement and of the co-design methodology was two-fold. Firstly, the students now had a specific space that they identified only with the therapeutic work and thus with the rules of the drama session as opposed to the rules of the classroom which allowed them to engage in the dramatherapy work more readily and with understanding about what was expected, allowed and not permitted. Because the space was physically and symbolically removed from their 'daily life' of the classroom where many of the issues that we were exploring (bullying, concentration, attention, group dynamics) originated from, these challenges were also put at a creative distance through the act of making a new space for them to work. This new space contributed to their group identity and contained the dramatherapy work.

Secondly, the act of appropriating and re-designing the space, setting up the curtain, chairs and lights through a co-design methodology contributed to this space becoming their own territory. Territoriality has since the dawn of time, been a privileged subject for interested ethologists and has become an object of study more or less central to a number of other disciplines including the human sciences via the notion of territory. Notions of territory have particularly interested a number of social and behavioural psychologists and psychoanalysts who argue that space is a structuring factor in the construction of identity. D.W. Winnicott understood very well the capacity of the environment to alter the meaning of things and to influence development and identity. With regards to child development, Winnicott proposed that a safe space co-constructs a solid and safe internal self-structure whereas a volatile, unpredictable and not 'good enough' environment can lead to a fractured or fragmented identity, emotional instability and even trauma.

Psychologist Jean Piaget, as part of his operational theory of intelligence, proposed a model linking the structuring of space and the construction of identity in children. Conceived as a psychic construction, the space favours the elaboration of the child's maturation processes and thus plays a central role in his emotional development and the construction of his Ego, or self. This idea was developed by social psychologist who emphasized the dynamic relationships between identity and territory, identity construction and the process of territorial appropriation.

Psychologist Lylian-Nemet Pier provides one theory on spatial appropriation and territory which supports this chapter's thesis that for space to be therapeutic it is most beneficial to design space *with* clients versus imposing space on clients or designing a space *for* them. In her article '*Investment and arrangement of the space and the family dynamic*' (2006) she argues that having access to a space to decorate engages the psychic process of projecting and forging one's inner self onto the blank canvas of the room which contributes to the development, reinforcement and communication of identity. In other words, *making* place affords a process of projection of a psychic self into reality. Moreover, appropriating a space contributes to a sense of territory, of 'ones-own-place', processes that are fundamental for the healthy development of children and adolescents in particular. Nemet-Pier associates the occupation of space with the theory of appropriation - which she describes as the personalization of space by an individual with precise and subjective marking behaviours – such as placing photos or rock posters on one's bedroom wall or in the case of my clients, creating decorative objects for the room and arranging the space together at the start of each session. The students took pride in cleaning the space before and after each session and over the course of the year, paintings, drawings and poetry adorned the walls and we could see the personality of each individual as well as the group in these spatial decorations. This contributed to a developing group identity and there was a tangible investment in the space which was reflected in their increased investment in the workshops. This process is not dissimilar to animals who mark their territories via sound or pheromone secretions as observed in studies in ethology. Nemet-Pier observes that in a personal space, such as the bedroom there is, in the best circumstances, on the one hand, the marking for oneself of one's own space: a corner of one's own with one's own objects and what should not be seen, a 'no man's land'. On the other hand, the marking of one's space becomes a signal for identity, the space becomes a place to show others what one's values are and makes it possible to display one's personality. The occupied space allows its inhabitant to affirm their identity, to express conflicts by arranging it in a certain way, to leave the imprint of their impulses (Nemet-Pier, 2006: 216–217). She describes how the impossibility of being able to appropriate space is often experienced as an abuse of power or domination over another or a group of others and can be felt as a negation of oneself from which the subject suffers. Having no space to call one's own has been linked to lower levels of self-esteem, an inability to thrive in education and an overbearing feeling of exclusion and diminished agency. Returning to theories of environmental psychology, I hypothesized that the absence of agency in their own home spaces (the inability to appropriate a corner of one's own) and even in the classroom upstairs (a space that was designed *for* the students as opposed to *with* them with layouts that were directed by norms in the antiquated French national education system) was perhaps part of the problem that contributed to the emergence of relational and behavioural conflicts in the individuals and in the group. Therefore, working with the space seemed an appropriate solution. Since this group, I have continued to observe children who come into my private practice and spend time adorning the walls with paintings or draping fabrics over the couch for the duration of their sessions, making it a little bit 'their own', even if for an hour each week.

## The curtain hides and reveals

The following example explores the presence of the theatre curtain in the dramatherapy space as a design object that becomes a vector for communication, containment, creativity and behavioural shifts.

In Greek mythology, Ariadne gave Theseus a ball of thread, called a *clew,* to facilitate his way out of her father's maze. From this myth gave rise to the use of the word *clew* to designate any tool that accompanies someone through difficulty. This signification eventually became understood as a piece of evidence that leads to a solution, and clew morphed into the modern English word, *clue*. In the following vignettes, it was the curtain, with its long green cotton threads stitched together to make a sheet, that became the initial *clew* as to the importance of the design of the therapy space and the object or furniture elements within which has guided me towards a spatial-thinking of dramatherapy ever since. I uphold the conviction that as drama therapists we must look to the clews implicit and explicit in the spaces within which we work, including the spatial objects, design objects, scenographies and architectures if you will, which play a leading role in the clinical and therapeutic work.

---

**Vignette Two**

The room is large and empty except for some chairs and tables pushed to the side and the long green curtain hanging from floor to ceiling, dividing the space in two with the intention to mark the distinction, separation or threshold between 'real life' and the 'imaginary world of play'. Julie is in dramatherapy for disruptive and violent behavioural tendencies.

I enter the room with the intention to facilitate a dramatherapy session centred on improvisation and role play. Julie ignores my invitation to sit in a circle on the floor for an opening ritual and instead rushes around the room like a tornado attempting to destroy anything she can in her path. She suddenly throws her body roughly onto the curtain that hangs quietly in the space.

Watching this interaction, I get the sense that the curtain is patiently waiting to welcome Julie's furore. Julie kicks the curtain with her feet then rips at the fabric with her hands trying, unsuccessfully, to pull it down then kicking it once more she runs and disappears behind it. The curtain remains in its place seemingly unbothered by the sudden physical and violent interaction, seamlessly shifting its role from punching bag to hidey-space in response to Julie's physical cues. Julie briefly reappears as if to check whether or not I am watching her, then she disappears once more with a roar of laughter. On the one hand, it seems to me that Julie is inviting me to play a game of hide-and-seek but on the other hand, her behaviour is an expression of defiance against the framework of the session: starting with a ritual in the circle on the floor. The curtain remains in its position and acts as a shield from my gaze. Tuning into what it tells me, I sense that Julie needs to spend some time hiding behind the curtain before dramatic play can occur, the curtain communicates to me that so early on in the dramatherapy work, perhaps Julie is not yet ready to trust. I notice that the curtain responds to Julie's needs by providing shelter, protection and concealment from view. Although, I find myself feeling curious as to her violence towards the curtain. The curtain-object, since the first moments of the session had only been present for her and supportive of her needs, was treated with such violence and rejection, and I speculate that while it may have simply been the only object in her war-path, I sense that there is deeper signification. I wonder if perhaps the curtain is me, or like-me. The curtain mirrors my intentions as a therapist: to be present, attentive and welcoming of all that Julie has to go through. While Julie doesn't dare kick me, she does dare to kick the curtain, a non-human but perhaps more-than-human object in the dramatherapy space. It is useful to view these spatial phenomena through a new-materialistic lens which I continue to develop in my thinking about place, space and dramatherapy, where new materialism's focus on materiality and bodily experience offers a way of contextualizing the coextensive relationship of the human self with the environment (Alaimo, 2010). I argue that the curtain object entered into this coextensive relationship that Stacey Alaimo talks about. I suggest that the curtain, which began as an inanimate object in the space, evolved into becoming what I saw as a co-therapist, taking on a life of its own to produce new meaning and creating new forms of agency in the space as well as supporting Julie in all the ways she needed it.

In another way, the curtain could be viewed as a *malleable medium* (Roussillon, 2001). The concept of malleable medium is developed by Roussillon from a hypothesis identified by Marion Milner (Brun, 2017). Roussillon purports that a malleable medium has five main properties: indestructibility, extreme sensitivity, indefinite transformation, unconditional availability and ability to perform on its own. The five elements can be described separately but their interdependence is essential for the malleable medium to take on its full value. The malleable medium appears as the transitional object and contributes to the process of representation. The malleable medium is internalized by the client, in the form of a *thing-representation*, and this contributes to organizing the secondary unconscious. In this previous vignette, I believe the curtain fulfilled this role of the malleable medium for Julie. It was available to receive Julie's physical aggressions onto its surface without being destroyed, it was sensitive in responding to her needs to be held returning a quality of care and softness due to its fabric makeup, it demonstrated its ability to be transformed (in the case of becoming a hammock), and was unconditionally available to Julie. Finally, it performs on its own by its presence in the room, offering a silent invitation of trust and a liminal and transitional space between *real* and *play* life.

**Vignette Three**

I have become accustomed to Julie's interactions with the curtain and I sense even more keenly that this developing child-to-object relationship is vital for her therapeutic progress. Therefore, employing an observational tool developed in my master's research thesis (Sweeney, 2015), I note down the ways in which she interacts with the curtain, at what moment in time it occurs in the session, followed by what is said or expressed physically and the frequency with which she interacts with the curtain, which facilitate my understanding of this object/space-to-client thera-peutic relationship. This has become 'The Object-to-Client Observation Scale' (Table 3.1). For each criterion, a mark out of five is attributed in order to calculate an average score attributed to each criterion. For more detailed information on this scale, see Sweeney, 2015.

I can see Julie's head poking out from one side of the curtain while the rest of her body is hidden from view. I wait quietly in the designated audience space. Quietly Julie slithers her body onto the stage space. She reminds me of a tired baby seal flopping about on the beach. She lethargically rolls towards the curtain and takes the long green cotton fabric trailing along the floor in her hands and slowly wraps her body tightly in the folds, resembling I note, something like a chrysalis. She is completely hidden in her curtain envelop and she remains there for a silent moment. For the first time in the year, words come and Julie tells me that she is in a 'hammock', and that she is 'dreaming', although she will not elaborate on her dream. Abruptly she unravels herself and jumps up in a burst of energy and laughter and returns to hide once more behind the curtain. The 'performance' is over and she comes out to take a bow.

This a big moment of firsts for Julie. Until now, Julie had not demonstrated an understanding of the separation between 'real life' and 'imaginative' life in the play space. Her bow signalled that she had perhaps understood the difference this time, that one moment on stage involved role play and the next moment, disappearing behind the curtain, was a moment of returning to herself. It was also the first time that the curtain facilitated and was involved in the creation of an imaginary world as opposed to being a receptacle for violence: a hammock and dream space. This recalls my description of the Freudian couch in the introduction to this volume. The couch promoted reverie and in the same way, the curtain object fulfilled a similar function, which in relationship to the curtain, Julie's inner life was played out. As Mannoni writes, 'when the curtain rises, it is the imaginary powers of the Self that are both released and organized' (Mannoni, 1969: 181).

Another first was that until this moment Julie had not put words on her experience on stage. French psychanalyst Patricia Attigui posits that the theatrical scene, and what relates to it, is to be seen as the necessary

*Table 3.1* The Object-to-Client Observation Table (Sweeney, 2015)

| | *Object: Curtain* | | | | |
|---|---|---|---|---|---|
| SCORE (*) | 1 | 2 | 3 | 4 | 5 |
| 1. Frequency | | | | | |
| 2. Priviledge | | | | | |
| 3. Symbolism | | | | | |
| 4. In which way was the object used | | | | | |
| Comments | | | | | |
| *Généralités* | | | | | |
| SCORE (*) | 1 | 2 | 3 | 4 | 5 |
| 5. Manifestation of aggression | | | | | |
| 6. Inhibition | | | | | |
| 7. Calme | | | | | |
| 8. Hyperactivity, agitation | | | | | |
| Comments | | | | | |
| *The Space* | | | | | |
| 9. Sound ambiance | | | | | |
| 10. Lighting | | | | | |
| 11. Temperature | | | | | |
| | *Object - Curtain* | | | | |
| SCORE (*) | 1 | 2 | 3 | 4 | 5 |
| 12. Behaviour, repetition, stereotypes | | | | | |
| 13. Anxiety | | | | | |
| 14. Overwhelmed by imagination | | | | | |
| 15. Delerium | | | | | |
| 16. Transgression: violence, acting out | | | | | |
| 17. Omnipotence | | | | | |
| Comments | | | | | |

Session Number:
Date:
Number of clients present:
Number of clients absents:
Name of client:
(*) Score
1: Not very frequently
2: A little frequently
3: Frequently
4: Very frequently
5: Always
*Note: Over a determined number of session, an average score attributed to each criterion can be calculated per client.*

framework for verbal elaboration (Attigui, 1993). This was evidenced here. It now seemed to me that Julie's relationship with the curtain was evolving from one of conflict to perhaps one of friendship and I wondered if she was perhaps feeling more accepting of or safe in her place in our therapeutic relationship as symbolized by this change in dynamic with the curtain. Moreover, I wondered if the act of wrapping and unwrapping herself had created a liminal space. As I mentioned earlier, she looked like a chrysalis, and jumping up I wondered, was she becoming a butterfly where this liminal space offered a place for transformation from one state to another? Whatever was occurring for Julie, the following months demonstrated a continued positive change in Julie's behaviour and creative process always in link with the curtain. Julie's violent and aggressive behaviour did not end entirely but she became more relaxed and less agitated and seemingly happier to come to her sessions.

### Vignette Four

Working with puppets this day, Julie chooses a boy puppet that she calls 'Zac'. Julie enters the stage space for a brief moment with 'Zac' before returning rapidly behind the curtain. She enters again and begins to play a family scene but quickly loses the thread of the narrative shifting from puppets to role play, herself embodying a monster character. Even though she still holds her marionette, it is not the puppet that is playing but Julie. Julie hits, bites and scratches the other puppet in the scene and she groans loudly. Julie throws her puppet across the room and launches herself at me. Following Julie's cues, a monster story pursues for a few moments until abruptly Julie stops playing, freezes and cries loudly, *'Stop! I'm scared!'* and she runs out of the room into the waiting room. The play ends. I follow Julie into the corridor. She is agitated and tells me she was scared of the monster. I sit with her till she is ready to return to the room. During this play, the world of imagination has taken on a real quality for Julie, and in that moment of fear she was unable to distinguish between play and reality. While Julie was unable to distinguish reality from fiction, what is remarkable in this vignette is the way in which, contrary to previous explosions of emotion (anger or fear specifically, where Julie would habitually hit or tear at the curtain) Julie did not project onto the curtain but rather was able to vocalize her fears in the words *'Stop! I'm scared'*.

It is the first time that Julie has been able to clearly identify her feelings with words rather than act out her fear through violence onto the curtain. Her response to run out of the room also marked a change in her relationship with the curtain where the curtain was no longer needed to contain her as it had before. I wondered if through her interactions with the curtain in previous months, Julie had internalized the symbolic function of the curtain, developing within herself a curtain-like psychic container that served to contain and support emotion.

In a reading of psychic containers, Didier Anzieu proposes through his skin-ego theory that in leaning onto the skin the psychic envelop continues, separates and organizes internal and external phenomena in the child (Anzieu, 1995, p. 85). Julie came from an inconsistent, unpredictable and disruptive home environment. In knowing this and observing Julie's aggressive behaviour coupled by her incapacity to contain or regulate her emotional self I argue that it may be possible that she began her therapy program with a fragile or porous skin-self as marked by emotional dysregulation, frustration intolerance, impulse control and acting-out. As Anzieu claims, where there is a fragile or porous self-ego the pare-excitement shield or protective psychic filter that wards off exogenous stimulus to provide a contained psychic space to regulate impulse and emotion, is at fault. Anzieu argues that in order to repair or reinforce this potentially fragile skin-ego, sensorial, tactile, kinesthetic, thermal and material contact with the skin is vital. This contact with the skin can also be understood from a reading of Donald Winnicott's theory of *holding, handling and object presenting* where the role of psychic maintenance is ensured by the internalization of appropriate holding and handling by the external environment which at the same time maintains and contains the whole of the child by continuously enveloping his body during its growth and development (Winnicott, 1971/2020). Winnicott's claim of a transitional object, the soft toy most often chosen by a small child, takes on this work of strengthening the self-ego through the soft fabric in contact with the child's skin in a similar way to Anzieu's theory. Thus, I suggest that Julie potentially found comfort in the soft cotton material of the curtain and that it was her physical and sensorial interaction with it, her enveloping and rubbing onto it that was the sensorial, tactile and haptic phenomenon needed in order to strengthen her fragile self-ego, emotional regulation and impulse control that reinforces both Anzieu and Winnicott's theories on space, object, materiality and self.

As the year approaches its end, Julie falls back into familiar habits of aggression and violence: hitting, kicking and tearing at the curtain once more. This regression of sorts is not surprising and appears to be the symptom of a deep separation anxiety that is being revived because of the closing therapy sessions. While this may appear to be a sign that things have not changed or progressed I am reassured by the fact that Julie is using a resource that she has refined over the course of the dramatherapy sessions: projecting onto the curtain, using it for safety, containment, creativity and care. Compared with the start of the year where Julie was not in control of her actions towards the curtain, in this instance it is very obvious that experiencing a heightened state of anxiety or anger, Julie takes the decision to express it towards the curtain. She is demonstrating that in moments of big emotion she knows that she is able to return to the curtain-object for support and that the curtain will offer her the support she needs. At the end of the final session, we passed from the stage space to the backstage side of the curtain, entering back into daily life and signifying the end of the therapeutic program.

## Discussion

In traditional theatre spaces with a proscenium arch, the curtain assists the scenography and marks the opening of the stage space, the unveiling of story. The curtain is the threshold between the real and imagined world. As we know, the etymology of theatre is the Greek *theatron*, a seeing place. At the moment of its opening the curtain and its game of *hide and reveal* are put into motion and serve to transport the viewer, or the player, into a fictitious world. It contributes to the unveiling of the world of the play, it hides and reveals literally as well as metaphorically

Through an environmental psychology-informed lens of space in dramatherapy, the design of a space dictates and guides movement and social interactions as well as impacting health, behaviour and relations. It guides relationships, movement and fosters transitions, it is affective, material and relational. Julie tested the safety of the therapeutic relationship through her engagement with the curtain and the game of hide and seek game. Her hiding communicated: Can you really *see* me? Will you find me or leave me? Is it safe to come out? Can I trust you? The curtain offered Julie a shield from my gaze, sensorial and tactile qualities and a liminal or threshold space between real and fictitious worlds. The curtain offered a 'seeing space' for Julie: a place to see and to be seen.

I suggest it can be useful to have a curtain in the dramatherapy room for two primary reasons. The first and most obvious is that it facilitates the magic 'as if' and the transition from 'real life' to 'imaginary life' for the client which is essential for dramatic play to occur. I have played with curtains, room dividers, Japanese folding doors, or the act of 'turning one's back to the audience' before revealing the character, but in all those experiments, the curtain was the most successful. Moving behind the curtain, the client is completely out of view from the gaze of the others in the group and/or therapist. Sometimes, of course, the therapist is behind the curtain with the client preparing to play together. Either way, this moment of concealment, of protection, can foster feelings of safety and can allow the client, like an actor before a show, to emotionally, psychologically and physically prepare to become *other*, literally and metaphorically.

The second meaning suggests that the curtain can be considered an actor in the space with an agentic power, as I have suggested could be viewed through a new materialistic lens. Art therapist Patricia Fenner reminds us that we must 'develop relationships not only with each other but also with material elements of the room for the purposes of support, and embrace place as constitutive in the event of therapy' (Fenner, 2011: 857). In my observations of the curtain, I argue that it fulfilled the following functions: a liminal space, a containing space, an envelope, a creative space and a relational function. I argue that the curtain demonstrated agentic qualities through its capacity to respond to Julie's emotional and relational needs. The curtain gave Julie a means through which to communicate, explore her imagination and creativity and contain and transform her emotional impulses. Furthermore, the curtain as an enveloping space absorbed the energetic and psychic impulses, such as fear and violence, that were otherwise unable to be psychically contained. In this way, the curtain took on the function of a potential and transitional object and space, providing a safe place through which to transition from fear to safety, from distance to proximity, from isolation to community and then at the end, through separation.

Through all the ways in which Julie played with the curtain as described above, the curtain shows itself to be anything but a passive object in the room. The curtain and Julie's relationship with it demonstrates an example of how the design elements in the dramatherapy room act or *do* all on their own. In viewing the curtain in this way provides an opportunity to consider *all* physical environments and the objects held within these therapeutic spaces as contributors to the therapeutic process in dramatherapy and beyond. As demonstrated, Julie used the curtain as an object of transfer, as an object of support, as a containing space for her overflowing impulses which contributed to the process of the construction of Self and iterates the notion that *where* we work, the design elements within the room we work, are essential to *what* happens and *how* therapy occurs.

## Conclusion

This chapter has intended to demonstrate the evolution of my thinking and practice with regard to the space, place, object, design and the built environment in dramatherapy. I have attempted to introduce the importance of making our session spaces *with* our clients as opposed to *for* them where co-creating offers a shared and agentic experience that reinforces identity, belonging, territory, safety, creativity, commitment to therapy and self-esteem. I have presented albeit briefly, the theorization of the curtain as a transitional space from a Winnicottian perspective and the curtain as contributing to a reinforced sense of self as scored by Anzieu's theories on skin-ego and psychic envelops, that can be explored through a sensorial and tactile encounter with the environment. I have also suggested that the curtain, as an example of specific objects in the built environment, as a malleable medium, becomes a co-therapist in the dramatherapy space.

The culmination of these experiences has led me to further investigate the potential impact of co-design practices *with* clients as a therapeutic practice. In the first example, feelings of territory led to a strengthening in group identity and engagement with the dramatherapy. For adults and children who have perhaps not had this opportunity or for whom that opportunity has been taken away due to institutionalization, appropriating the dramatherapy space can establish a feeling of having a space of one's own, of feeling at home, as well as projecting and communicating their individual and group identities into the physical space of the session making it a psycho-social space. I argue that it is essential that we consider the therapeutic spaces in institutions and consider the possibilities and ways of appropriating these shared spaces for mental health benefits. A dramatherapy setting can provide a creative opportunity to spend time making space with our clients, in order to give them a place of their own, facilitate and promote group identity and dynamics, and increase individual self-esteem and agency over their therapeutic program. In support of this Patricia Fenner has argued that

> [t]he notion of the therapy room as place, as a component in the "spatiality of care", illuminates its value as a material and expressive event; one which more inclusively attends to the forces and relationships within the room, including rich encounters being made with objects and zones and the meaning-making processes, which transpire.
>
> (Fenner, 2011, p. 851)

Today, designing *with* versus designing *for* is central to my dramatherapy practice and identity as a drama therapist and I have continued to wonder: what impact does arranging and making space with clients have on their sense of agency over their therapeutic process? What choices are made about spatial configuration and appropriation and what do these choices result in? In co-designing the space with the children, I sought to co-construct a 'good enough' therapeutic space that supports the internal landscapes that were being encountered in the dramatherapy space. Offering a good enough environment for our clients in dramatherapy does not assume that the environment is perfect but it becomes a question of our ethical positioning as therapists whereby awareness and attunement into the spaces within which our clients encounter themselves and the other is vital for best practice.

I have since pushed this idea of making and designing space *with* clients towards the shaping and building of huts, tents, caverns, nests, etc. in the dramatherapy room, that sees place making as an art therapeutic medium, of which I described a few short examples. Making tents and huts goes beyond simply shifting furniture and proposes an artistic technique to address agency, self-esteem, identity and inner landscapes. Further insight into the process of making huts and tents and the therapeutic impact of that artistic process can be found in a reading of my chapter 'A Space of their Own: A case-study advocating appropriation of the domestic interior for well-being' in *Interiors in the Era of Covid-19* (Sweeney and Messer, 2022).

Successful or not in my claims, my main purpose of this chapter is to spark debate and discussion around why and how we design therapeutic space, to promote understanding of objects as powerful actors in the therapy space, and to reflect upon what our working environments *do*. I am currently pursuing a doctoral research project in Architecture and the Built Environment. At the heart of engaging space as a medium for therapeutic outcomes is the understanding that 'we shape ourselves by shaping the world' (Levine, 2020: 3) and inversely that shaping worlds, shapes selves. I argue that the practice of shaping place and space in any therapeutic context demands an explicit understanding of the effect of space on the psychology, behaviour and emotions of individuals and groups. This chapter is a small window into the many possibilities that space and place can affect dramatherapy process and I conclude with a call for increased explicit attention toward the therapeutic impact of designing *with* clients across interdisciplinary practices.

## References

Alaimo, S. (2010) *Bodily Natures: Science, Environment, and the Material Self.* Bloomington: Indiana University Press.

Anzieu, D. (1995) *Le Moi-Peau.* Paris: Dunod (Psychismes).

Attigui, P. (1993) *De L'illusion Théâtrale à L'espace Thérapeutique: Jeu, Transfert et Psychose.* Paris: Denoël (L'Espace analytique).

Barker, R. (1968). *Ecological Psychology : Concepts and Methods for Studying the Environment of Human Behavior.* Palo Alto, CA, USA: Stanford University Press.

Brun, A. (2017) 'Les Médiations Thérapeutiques', *Canal Psy*, 120, pp. 10–13. Available at: 10.35562/canalpsy.1798

Crang, M, and Thrift, N. J. (eds.) (2000). *Thinking Space.* New York:Routledge.

Fenner, P. (2011) 'Place, Matter and Meaning: Extending the Relationship in Psychological Therapies', *Health & Place*, 17(3), pp. 851–857. Available at: 10.1016/j.healthplace.2011.03.011

Fordham, M. (1978). *Jungian Psychotherapy. A Study in Analytical Psychology.* New York, NY:Wiley.

Grainger, R. (2003) 'We'Ll Hang Ourselves Tomorrow - "Waiting for Godot" as Therapeutic Theatre', *Dramatherapy*, 25(2), pp. 17–18. Available at: 10.1080/02630672.2003.9689628

Hocini, F., Le Run, J.-L., and Potel Baranes, C. (2006). De l'espace avant toute chose. *Enfances & Psy*, 33(4), pp. 610.3917/ep.033.0006.

Levine, S.K. (2020) 'Ecopoiesis: Towards a Poietic Ecology'. Available at: 10.24412/2713-184X-2020-1-17-24

Lingiardi, V. and De Bei, F. (2011) 'Questioning the Couch: Historical and Clinical Perspectives', *Psychoanalytic Psychology*, 28(3), pp. 389–404. Available at: 10.1037/a0024357

Mannoni, O. (1969) *Clefs Pour L'imaginaire, Ou L'autre Scène.* Paris: Editions du Seuil.

Nemet-Pier, L. (2006) 'Investissement et Aménagement de L'espace Dans la Dynamique Familiale', *Imaginaire & Inconscient*, 18(2), p. 215. Available at: 10.3917/imin.018.0215

Proshansky, H. M. (1976). 'Environmental Psychology and the Real World', *American Psychologist*, 31, 303–310. 10.1037/0003-066x.31.4.303

Proshansky, H., Ittelson, W., and Rivlin, L. (Eds). (1970). *Environmental Psychology: Man and His Physical Setting.* New York: Holt:Rinehart and Winston.

Roussillon, R. (2001) 'L'objet « Médium Malléable » et la Conscience de soi:', *L'Autre*, 2(2), pp. 241–254. Available at: 10.3917/lautr.005.0241

Sanders, J. (ed.) (2020) *Stud: Architectures of Masculinity*. 1st edn. London: Routledge.

Sommer, R., and Olsen, H. (1980). 'The Soft Classroom', *Environment and Behavior*, 12( 1), pp. 3–16. 10.1177/0013916580121001

Sweeney, E. & Messer, S. (2022) 'A Space of their Own: A Case-Study Advocating Appropriation of the Domestic Interior for Well-Being', in Scholze, J. *et al.* (ed.) (2022) *Interiors in the Era of COVID: Interior Design between the Public and Private Realms*. 1st edn. London [England]: Bloomsbury Visual Arts.

Sweeney, E. (2015) 'L'Espace Théatro-Thérapeutique', Paris Descartes University: Unpublished Master's Thesis: https://www.academia.edu/44358408/Master_1_ Research_Thesis_a_study_of_the_therapeutic_impact_of_the_theatre_and_sceno-graphic_space_on_children_in_paediatric_psychiatry_in_a_dramatherapy_setting

Warf, B. and Arias, S. (eds.) (2014) *The Spatial Turn: Interdisciplinary Perspectives*. 1. Issued in Paperback. London: Routledge (Routledge studies in human geography, 26).

Winnicott, D.W. (2020) *Jeu et Réalité: L'espace Potentiel*. Translated by C. Monod and J.-B. Pontalis. Paris: Gallimard.

Wong, C., Sommer, R., and Cook, E. (1992). 'The soft classroom 17 years later,' *Journal of Environmental Psychology*, 12(4), pp. 337–343.

# 4 Neutral Mask and Embodied Dreamwork, Spaces of Containment

*Mayra Stergiou*

This chapter aims to stress the emerging practice of Embodiment and the Neutral Mask in Dramatherapy and will present a group case study of the use of the Neutral mask to investigate the impact on male offenders in prison and offer practical insights into the applications of these theatre-derived techniques. In particular, it aims to draw attention to the use of J. Lecoq's Neutral Mask as a containing space of the inner reality and self-expression of the client, within the context of Dramatherapy practice. It will shed light on the therapeutic potential of working with dreams and images through embodiment work and the use of the mask. This chapter finally aims to demonstrate how this work has been adapted from the performer's training to the dramatherapeutic space to fit the needs of psychological healing. Within the dramatherapy sessions in a prison context, I bridge two practices: the work of Jacques Lecoq's Neutral Mask traditionally used in the context of performance making with professional actors and Embodied Dreamwork that derives from the Jungian Psychoanalyst Robert Bosnak. Both dream and mask spaces are central to my approach in dramatherapeutic work. The influence of Jacques Lecoq on modern theatre is significant but his practice has been little explored within dramatherapy therefore, I will cover a brief history of its origins and use and then demonstrate how it was applied to male prison offenders. The chapter will detail some exercises used and methods applied in the creation of therapeutic spaces with neutral mask and dreamwork. I argue that the symbolic and essentially scenographic spaces of embodied dream work in combination with Neutral Mask space in dramatherapy contain powerful emotional states and facilitate resilience and provoke change and healing within the prison context.

## Jacques Lecoq Theatre Training

J. Lecoq founded an international school of performance training in Paris in 1956 at which he taught until a few days before his death in 1999. Many of his past students have gone on to form their own devised companies, such as Le Théâtre du Soleil, Complicite, Mummenschantz and many others worldwide. Graduates have also found success as theatre and film actors and directors

DOI: 10.4324/9781003252399-6

(e.g. Geoffrey Rush, Julie Taymor, Luc Bondy, Simon McBurney). Lecoq's guiding principle was *tout bouge* – everything moves. His rigorous analysis of movement in humans and their environments formed the foundation for a refined and nuanced repertoire of physical exercises. These exercises, including the work with the Neutral Mask, develop a heightened somatic awareness of the actor and their relationship between thought, feeling, gesture and language, preparing them to communicate with movement in a variety of styles, to employ physical actions that both provoke and define emotion and to invest spoken language with meaningful gesture. Parts of these exercises have been integrated as part of the dramatherapy sessions with male offenders that this chapter will detail in later parts.

The Neutral Mask is a full-face leather mask with a neutral facial expression. It is neither joyful nor sad, angry nor determined. Its expression is indiscernible and in a variety of dramatic exercises as well as observing others doing the same, wearing this mask permits actors to develop a heightened awareness of the communicative potential of the body and, thus, access heightened states of self-awareness and sensorial phenomenon, as defined by Lecoq as the 'poetic body'. Neutral Mask work in Dramatherapy focuses the attention of the client immediately on movement and engages the involvement of physical activity with physical communication. Since we often pay great attention to facial expressions in daily life, the communicative content of posture, gesture and gait becomes much more apparent to the observer when the face is covered by the mask – information that can then be used in the dramatherapy sessions. Employing the Neutral Mask in a therapeutic context can allow the participants to get in touch with their bodies at a sensorial level, to be fully present and to allow powerful emotions, images and memories to be expressed through the safe container of the mask space as well as the embodied structure of their inner dream images.

Lecoq's use of the mask to train actors is prescient of the discoveries within cognitive science in many ways. For example, by heightening an actor's awareness and expressive control of postural communication, Lecoq's Neutral Mask exercises assist in clarifying emotional expression when the mask is removed (Lecoq used the Neutral Mask only in training, not for performance). For the dramatherapy client who enters the mask space, an interesting phenomenon arises as one doesn't need to concern oneself with facial expression as the primary means of communication, prolonged use of the mask encourages relaxation of the facial muscles that in turn seems to prompt a sense of calm and focus. This was observed within dramatherapy sessions in the forensic prison setting. This approach diminishes the focus of the client to create conscious cognitive facial expressions of a character or of its dream images, which is often focused on language and intellectual cognition and consequently allows unconscious and embodied images to emerge leading towards a more authentic expression resulting in creating an abstract yet truthful and potentially healing construction. Psychologist Paul Ekman's work on facial expressions has shown that consciously arranging the facial musculature in the patterns associated with various primary emotions provokes the affective state of the emotion. This indicates that there is a reflexive proprioceptive relationship between facial musculature and emotion, a phenomenon that may explain the sense of calm that arises from the relaxation of the facial muscles under the mask. Other researchers point to a similar reflexive (or reciprocal) relationship between larger bodily activity and the experience of emotion. Movement of the whole body is involved in Neutral Mask identification work, in which the wearer of the mask consciously embodies the rhythms of movement found in natural, social and fabricated environments. In contact with movement, the environment around becomes a dream space and encourages images to arise from the dream narratives, simultaneously accessing the unconscious. This activity forms the foundation of the remarkable synchrony between Lecoq's pedagogy and the precepts of embodied cognition. It articulates Lecoq's conviction that the starting point for theatre is not a scripted play but rather the actor's engagement with the sensorimotor experience of their environment. Beginning with sensorimotor investigations and moving through spoken than written language, Lecoq's training grounds performance in an explicit re-experiencing of human cognitive development. In Dramatherapy, this re-experiencing can be very useful for the client to get in touch with memories that could not be accessible in traditional verbal psychotherapy or too painful to address with words. Following this experience in the dramatherapy setting, the client is invited to create a free association piece of writing based on the experience he/she had wearing the mask and then, to embodying the inner landscapes of their imagination. The reflections that might come out of such process are expressed in the use of an 'inner landscape' where the client becomes the architect of his inner life and imagination and having the agency to create the changes that need to be made and reclaim their lost narratives.

### Embodied Imagination

The work with dreams and images within dramatherapy, is influenced by the theory of Embodied Imagination of Robert Bosnak. According to Bosnak, the activity of dreams, as natural and innate as the human heartbeat, has extraordinary therapeutic potential and is widely thought to trigger the body's own self-healing response (2007). When we pay unbiased attention to our dreams, we notice that we are in a world where multiple perspectives coexist. Dreams appear as self-manifestations of landscapes, environments, people, animals and a variety of other presences such as traffic lights and kitchen sinks. Embodied Imagination theory approves Freud's view that dreams are unconscious representations but challenges the notion that dreams are merely disguises of desires (Zhen-Dong, Wang Baohong and Qian, 2020). Using the physical body as the work anchor point and the reaction container, emphasizing the function of emotions and feelings appeared in the dream, and reinterpreting the synchronization and transference between the therapist and the client. Building community allows participants to feel safe enough to take risks together by using embodied interventions. Jones (2007) defined embodiment, or physical participation, as one of the core processes of dramatherapy (Jones, 2007: 112). Embodied techniques include sculpting, mirroring, role enactment, role-play and developmental transformations, during which attention is paid to the body. The body becomes the space that consists of the inner landscapes of the emotional and sensorial experiences, the memories, the traumas and the untapped potentialities of change. Interesting to note, J. Lecoq's method is situated alongside the theories of analytical psychology of C.G. Jung which also gave birth to the Embodied Dramaturgy approach of Thomas Prattki in Berlin in 2017. Prattki's Embodied Dreamwork approach, within a theatrical context, is based on creating a theatre of images that arises from the performer's body after a process of individuation and working with and through myths, improvisations, tales, fantasy novels and contemporary paintings as a point of departure. Performers are invited to explore the fears and fantasies of the collective unconscious as C.G Jung defined it around the inner shadowlands and inner landscapes (Jung, 1959). This artistic approach also involves use of Theatre of Images, Object Theatre, Puppetry and the Theatre of the space of the fantastical. Theatre of Images places the focus on frozen images using the performer's body to respond to a given stimulus such as words or a phrase. These frozen images act as a catalyst for discussion. They offer an opportunity to access a diverse range of responses which can be explored without necessarily being bound by the language, jargon, culture and expectations of the performer before the rehearsal begins. Performers might be invited to bring their own dreams or work with spontaneous reflections in a discussion circle before the physical warm-up. Embodied dreamwork in a therapeutic context uses the client's body to anchor the feelings arising from the space of the dream images. In other words, the body becomes the locus for the emotional experience of the dream. The dreamwork is experienced in a hypnagogic state, a state between sleep and wakefulness. During the dreamwork, the dreamer is asked to focus on the multiple sensations arising from the images. The dreamworker, or therapist, serves as a coach, asking the dreamer questions to help amplify the dream images. The technique is not interpretative. Rather, it supports the dreamer in linking sensory experiences of the dream to corresponding affective and somatic states. Other physicalized experiences create space for discovery. Embodied dreamwork further resembles movement therapy in that movement can be internal when the dreamers concentrate on an affective state, or external when dreamers make involuntary movements in response to feelings.

## Case Study

In 2008 and 2009, I was working as a trainee dramatherapist at a Category B therapeutic community within a prison service in the United Kingdom. A group of male inmates were referred to join a weekly dramatherapy group as part of their participation in the therapeutic community of verbal psychotherapies program. This was the first pilot arts therapies project within the service, aimed at offering an alternative to verbal psychotherapies. Drama-based methods which have been based on the CBT framework are The Mask (Baim, Brookes and Mountford, 2002), Role Theory and Role-Play (Moreno, 1962). In this program, the model used was the integrative dramatherapy model and aspects of systemic and psychoanalytic framework were also influencing the theoretical framework of the sessions. The program was designed to promote wellbeing, enable anger management and strengthen communication and relational skills between members and the staff. The sessions also focused on tapping into the collective and individual creative potential and the rehabilitative process of the members of being allowed the opportunity to express feelings in a way that is helpful to them. The members were referred to the dramatherapy group either as a complementary to the group psychotherapy or due to difficulties with emotional expression and self-disclosure. Inmates initially attended individual dramatherapy assessment sessions where they revealed negative experiences with prison life, perceived repression, anxiety, fear, emotions related to deprivation and the loss of relationships, former participation to gangs, substance use problems, sleep deprivation and re-occurring nightmares.

Specifically, the aims of the dramatherapy program were to:

- Strength the resilience of the group and build self-confidence
- The group members were invited to come up with their own individual and group goals and revise them with the completion of the sessions
- Mediation and grounding - noticing what is going on in mind and body, letting go of anxieties and tension, bringing focus into the session
- Though the embodiment of dreams, images and the enactment of stories the group was encouraged to become in touch with the space of their imagination while remaining focused on the present
- To relate to dissonant and harmonious parts of themselves, to open themselves and to tolerate ambiguity, and not narrowing to polarities and make conscious connections and meaning making of the dreams by associating dream elements to life events
- To feel, express and work through difficult emotions and build containment and safety in themselves and in relation to others

The structure of each session was separated into 4 stages taken from the Sesame Dramatherapy Structure:

- Warm Up: breath work/check in the here and now)
- Bridge In: any connections with the previous session/ a dream or an image to narrate in the circle)
- Enactment: the participants who would be willing to embody aspects of the dream or the whole dream as a story and one member or more than one would be invited to wear the mask and embody the images)

- Bridge Out: de-rolling the space of the enactment, taking off the mask and or verbalizing anything towards the mask/characters as separate objects
- Warm down/ Closure: return to the circle and sharing, making any connections with reality in the here and now

Members met weekly in a room with transparent glass windows. From the beginning, this space influenced the theme of the first group session, as the lack of privacy became an issue to explore with the inmates. Questions and feelings around blurred boundaries between the private and the public, what is seen and what remains unexposed, gave birth to another space. This space was located in the dramatherapeutic space itself that needed to be defined anew by the members reclaiming their capacity to 'define' their personal space within the prison and consequently to locate it within themselves. The group decided to use fabrics from my dramatherapy box to cover the windows as part of creating and owning their own safe space within the room. However, this activity contradicted the rules and regulations of the prison and was therefore discontinued. The group decided then to focus on ways to create 'safe' spaces within the sessions and the space they were in that did not contradict the prison rules. Each member used fabrics, chairs and objects available in the session to create their own individual 'safe spaces'. Then as if in a museum, the group was invited to visit everyone's safe space. In this work, members of the group explored themes of personal space versus public space, individual spaces versus group spaces and boundaries. Below, I am going to describe some aspects of the dramatherapy sessions.

The aim of the first four sessions was for each member to introduce themselves and establish trust in the group. The sessions always began with breath work and tai-chi exercises for relaxation as most members mentioned suffering from stress and anxiety during the initial assessments. Members came to dramatherapy sessions with high levels of anxiety and reoccurring nightmares. Before the mask work and the dream enactments could begin, we focused on reflections from the previous sessions and moved into movement and rhythm of breath. Breath work enabled the group to express the images that were coming to them more freely while they were narrating their dreams.

The members were invited to create an imaginary box and to place their names inside thus introducing the members from very early on to the language of imaginary and projective play. The boxes were in microscale and the members used their hands to create them. The box became the first space to contain each personal story of the members symbolized in their names. According to Timothy Baima and Michael E. Sude, 'this activity can facilitate self-reflection, group bonding and play an important role in demonstrating values of equity and social justice' (Baima and Sude, 2020: 1–22). The group was invited to bring a dream and/or an image of a dream to the sessions. This invitation arose after a couple of the members started bringing their dreams into the session and reported issues with nightmares and difficulties with sleeping. writes that metaphor is now generally accepted as a fundamental mode of cognition and not simply a figure of speech or a feature of language. He defines metaphor, in part, as a transfer or moving of meaning between dissimilar domains; this transfer acknowledges the play of similarity and difference. In the work of Embodied Dreamwork this may be understood thus: as the client embodies the dream image through empathic identification—that is, as she or he enters the image and feels it in the body—the patient is employing an open and fluid use of metaphor. During the dreamwork, she or he enters many different types of images but remains oneself at the same time, experiencing a dual consciousness, a sense of similarity while maintaining difference. Mancia (2006) cites neuroscientific and psychoanalytic support for the hypothesis that implicit memories store the early emotional and affective, at times traumatic, pre-symbolic and preverbal experiences of the primary mother-infant dyad. In his view, they form the early, unrepressed unconscious nucleus of the self. Although formed very early, these memories can condition the affective, emotional, cognitive and sexual life of the adult. However, although these memories create lasting patterns, they are also plastic and can change. They can be reprocessed, recontextualized, and transformed to create new patterns or schemas (Edelman, 1987).

I observed that one of the dreams that a member brought to the group during the last few sessions of work together was the image of a grieving woman, who peels potatoes and spends her life in the desert waiting to die. When she dies, the woman goes to paradise where she is reunited with loved ones and other members of her family. The client ties a black fabric to his head and asks the group to accompany him with drums as he is singing in the desert. After having been absent for several sessions, this was the first time the inmate played with the group. At the end, he shakes the imaginary sand out of his body and sits in the circle. In the following session, he brings a personal object with him and shares it with the group. He speaks about his last memories with his mother. He remarks that one of the most painful moments in his life – despite the gangs, and his crimes – was the moment he was invited to play again, in the dramatherapy session. He notes that it was painful because he could not remember how to begin playing. He explained that this unknowing of how to play was his reason for leaving the group in the first place. As we worked through the dream image of the desert with the singing, the importance of the 'absent' space of play became a powerful metaphor. Gradually, the surviving, exhausted habitual self was less in evidence and replaced with more vitality and confidence along with increased creativity. I wonder if the early unconscious 'knowing' of the victimized self-altered and changed to become a more playful, trusting and spontaneous self.

From sessions 4–8, as the group became more familiar with both the artistic medium of the dramatherapy sessions and with each other and we moved into the phase of enactment of dreams and the embodiment of images through the use of the Neutral Mask. The group was initially introduced to the Neutral Mask as an 'object'. The members were invited to observe the mask, to pass the mask around the circle and explore the texture, shape and figurative characteristics of the mask. A brief introduction to the history of the mask had been provided by the workshop facilitator in the prison and the members were invited to verbalize their first spontaneous thoughts or questions they had in reaction to the mask as they were passing them around. One reaction was a common issue noted among the inmates which was a felt need to 'put on a mask' in order to survive in often-intimidating environments, such as prison. The members of the group voiced their belief that projecting an aggressive demeanor would help them in potentially difficult situations. As such, issues with aggressiveness could become ingrained in their personality. Gradually opening themselves to 'the space of the mask' during the dramatherapy sessions revealed aspects of the unconscious inner life of the participants, such as this need to wear a mask or aggressive demeanors, unknown up to this point, and enabled them to bring to the surface a more integrated whole. According to Robert Landy, 'the mask, although not attached to the face, is an object of minimal distance, because when worn it becomes part of the face' (Landy, 1996a: 13). It is, however, more distancing than makeup as it can be removed easily and referred to as a separate entity in the therapy session. The mask is used as a projective device. It is an image of the transcendent part of the human being, that which strives toward a more perfect existence and battles with deep-rooted fears. In therapy, the mask is an image of the self. The external focus of theatre takes a turn inward in therapy. The godlike, emblematic, universal quality of the mask points not to the head and the heavens, but to the heart' (Landy, 1985: 7).

Following the introduction to the mask, the inmates were invited to wear a mask and focus on the sensory elements of the mask against their skin. Then they were invited to focus on a single part of the body for example, the arms, or the right-hand fingers and one at a time and in slow rhythm to move them. They were then invited to focus on the whole hand, then the wrist, the elbow and finally the shoulder, moving up and around the body till the whole self had been visited. These exercises occurred in pairs and the members were invited to mirror each other. We employed mimesis, which is understood here to mean 'the compulsion to become like other' (Auerbach & Said, 2003 ). Using this mimetic dramatic craft, allowed the inmates to be taken over by the characters of their dreaming. In this way, they ended up in an embodied world of multiple characters existing simultaneously. Each character had its own perspective. Becoming aware of them as a potential state of consciousness has dramatic results. Allowing the routine experience of the inmates through the dramatherapy work, allowed them to interact with non-self-experiences and leave behind the condition in which they are the protagonists on the stage of life involved in deafening self-hypnotic monologues.

As we dialogued with 'what's different' from our habitual states of consciousness, we become a self-organizing system without an overarching controlling self. In the act of wearing the mask, it was intended that the members of the group would experience the elimination of the conception of time and of normally shared space, which afforded them the opportunity to go inside themselves, to face their own fears, spontaneous thoughts, images and senses that might occur in that moment. Everyone was sitting on the ground, legs crossed, the torso bent over so that the head rested on the legs. Wearing the mask, members of the group were invited to slowly start waking up parts of their bodies, fingers, toes, etc. until they moved to standing, gradually proceeding to walk. The inmates were invited to imagine that they see a light and to follow that light to a cave where they believe to have been sleeping for 100 years. Finally, inmates were invited to leave the cave and hold onto the first imagination image they had after they left the cave. In the next session, members were invited to embody these imagination images that they encountered at the exit of the cave. The images that members brought were varied from more abstract to concrete, images from childhood memories to animals. The awakening of the mask and the embodiment of the images after the cave was the first contact with the notion of metaphor and an attempt of building empathy towards the image and the parts of the self that might be fragmented due to the histories of traumas that members brought in the assessment sessions. Domash remarks that '[t]his practice challenges and expands the "habitual self," considered part of the repetition compulsion, accomplished, in part, by reaching the underlying metaphoric processes involved in imagination' (Domash, 2016: 21). A key part of a rehabilitative process for inmates involves being offered the opportunity to express feelings in a way that is helpful to them. During a mid-evaluation of the programme with staff members, participants were reported to have reduced feelings of anger and some reduction in incidents of physical aggression. The focus on the embodied experiences of the members in contrast with discussion-based approaches, used in mandatory treatment programmes are often futile attempts to rehabilitate as many patients find it difficult to talk about their problems when asked.

Working creatively with offenders in prisons has been shown to bring about constructive change. However, some would still raise the question as to whether 'drama can contribute significantly to that process of change' (Etherton and Prentki, 2006: 24–28). In the sessions that follow, members went deeper into the embodiment of dream images and group processes started to unfold. The sessions had a mixture of improvisation games and play in every warm-up in order to facilitate an atmosphere of playfulness and openness to prepare the work for the difficult and painful at times emotions explored. During this phase of group development, two members left the group. Whilst some members were drawn by the metaphors and images of their dreams, others they were interested to bring more realistic parts of their lives and place they had once inhabited. During the enactments, connections between the members would be facilitated and encouraged to use role reversals and being in each other's images to facilitate empathy. The memories and stories of the members have been incorporated into the embodied dream process. The work with the mask has also deepened at this stage of the process. The inmates were gradually taking more risks in their enactments using the mask. We also used aspects from the embodiment of the Neutral Mask

Journey from J. Lecoq physical theatre training but adapted to the needs of the dramatherapy space. For example, the members were invited to walk through a dense forest and climb a mountain. They were invited to do the same exercise wearing the mask and then without. From this stage, gradually the members were encouraged to embody images at their choice of wearing or not wearing the mask depending on their comfort zone of self-expression. At times the mask became another character in the room that they were able to remove from their face and directly speak to them. In this way, the members were invited to gradually take distance from the embodied selves and possibly externalize the internal dialogues and become more conscious of the existence of these different stories towards a more integrated self. One of the members of the group wanted to enact a real story of a disagreement with a staff member. Usually, I would encourage the members to stay within the boundaries of the metaphor, however, this felt a significant moment for this particular member. We used three chairs and the role reversal exercise from the psychodrama techniques to facilitate empathy with the 'other' and looking at the conflict from different perspectives.

During the final sessions, the members were invited to transform the room into their personal landscape and create an individual map of their journeys during the dramatherapy group. The members were given time at this stage to gradually integrate their imaginary stories and dream images into their reality and make connections with their current issues and life in prison. The Neutral Mask also became a space of letting go of anything they wanted to leave behind and/or didn't want to carry with. During the last sessions, the members were no longer using the mask but used the same principles expanded to the spaces they were creating. The 'mask' has become the spaces of their enactments. At the end of the journey, one for the members, the youngest in the group (21 years old) that had been predominantly engaging with the reality of his personal stories and who had difficulty in engaging with metaphor and imaginative play space, drew a picture of a home. He later asked me if I could take the drawing out of the prison and throw it into a river, seeing as he could not go out of the prison himself. The space of the mapping became a significant metaphor for his own life and his desire for freedom and feelings of despair. We agreed to complete this ritual within the boundaries of the dramatherapy session. As a trainee facilitator, this also signified a breakthrough in my development as a therapist. I had to be aware and reflect on my own desire to 'save' the client versus my role as a dramatherapist and bring these insights as countertransference back to the therapy session.

Part of the embodied mask work was to enable inmates with histories of violence and violent outbursts to consider their roles in society, build up their repertoire of skills, experience the range of their emotions and come in touch with other parts of relating and responding to the world around them by responding to the spaces within them. Role Theory suggests that learning how to perform and adapt to different roles in life is an important life skill' (Landy, 1996b: 223). Also, Baim and Mountford suggest that '[i]f the participant is motivated, they can use role-play to help develop the thinking skills, the inter-personal skills and the confidence to make the changes they want to make' (Baim, Brookes and Mountford, 2002).

## Conclusion

In this chapter, I set out to describe how the use of the space of embodied dream work in combination with Neutral Mask work meets in dramatherapy with male offenders in a prison context to explore the inner reality and self-expression of the workshop participants. The use of drama-based methods as a form of rehabilitation for offenders has been assessed and proven to provide ways for inmates to re-learn how to become contributing, valued members of society while understanding how to change the negative aspects of themselves that led to their offending behavior (Osborn-Greatrex, 2018, 19). Feedback collected from the staff who were involved in this project indicated that parti-cipants were able to increase their motivation to change and to develop insight and skills needed to effectively engage with others. By talking through their feelings using the mask the participants could analyze their own behavior. Inmates relayed the difficulties they faced in the sessions through having to open up in session, use projective play, in accessing their playfulness and emotional expression. Overall, positive emotions were communicated, and the most dis-cussed theme that was highlighted from within the project was the motivation to change. Bromberg writes that the therapeutic relationship can be thought of as 'a journey in which two people must each loosen the rigidity of their disso-ciative "truths" about self and other to allow "imagination" to find its shared place' (Bromberg, 2013: 3). Even though early implicit memories are set down neurologically, recent practice and research have demonstrated that memory is plastic and can be recontextualized and given new meaning (Bruhn, 1990: 95–104). If this process is open and fluid, we can view the past from the per-spective of our adult and more integrated self and create new meanings and perceptions working through the fragmentations of early traumatic experiences. As the inmates re-entered the dream space during the enactment, I noticed that they became more relaxed, less aggressive and playful with their imagination. Overall, although drama-based interventions in prisons haven't been without its criticism, this approach could offer a way forward drawing upon the neutral mask within the dramatherapy setting to enhance inmates' wellbeing, education and mental health and to contribute complementary to verbal psychotherapies rehabilitation programs.

## References

Auerbach, E. and Said (2003) Mimesis: The Representation of Reality in Western Literature - Fiftieth-Anniversary Edition Paperback – July 1, Princeton Classics

Baima, T., Michael and Sude, E. (2020) 'The Whole Name Exercise: A Self of the Therapist Activity to Support Culturally Attuned and Inclusive Communities in MFT Training, May 2020', *Journal of Family Psychotherapy*, 32(1), pp. 1–22

Baim, C., Brookes, S., and Mountford, A. (2002) *The Geese Theatre Handbook: Drama with Offenders and People at Risk*. Waterside Press.

Bosnak, R. (2007) *Embodiment: Creative Imagination in Medicine, Art and Travel*. New York, NY: Routledge.

Bromberg, P.M. (2013) 'Hidden in Slain sight: Thoughts on Imagination and the Lived Unconscious', *Psychoanal. Dial.*, 23, pp. 1–14.

Bruhn, A.R. (1990) 'Cognitive-perceptual theory and the projective use of autobiographical memory'. *Journal Pers Assess*. 1990 Fall;55(1-2), pp. 95–114.

Domash, L. (2016). Dreamwork and Transformation: Facilitating Therapeutic Change Using Embodied Imagination. *Contemporary Psychoanalysis*, 52, 410–43310.1080/00107530.2016.1198885

Etherton, M. and Prentki, M. '"Drama for change? Prove it! Impact assessment in applied theatre." (2006): Research in Drama Education', *The Journal of Applied Theatre and Performance*, 11, pp. 139–155.

Jones, P. (2007) *Drama as Therapy Volume 1: Theory, Practice and Research*, 2nd ed. London: Routledge.

Jung, C.G. (1959 [1944]) *Psychology and Alchemy: CW Vol 12. Trans. R.F.C. Hull. New edition.* London: Routledge and Kegan Paul.

Landy, R.J. (1996a) *The Couch and the Stage: Integrating Words and Actions in Psychotherapy*. Lanham, MD: The Rowman & Littlefield Publishing Group, Inc.

Landy, R.J. (1996b) *Essays in Drama Therapy: The Double Life*. Jessica Kingsley.

Landy, R. (1985) 'The Image of the Mask: Implications for Theatre and Therapy', *Journal of Mental Imagery*, 9(4), pp. 43–56.

Mancia, M. (2006).'Implicit Memory and Early Unrepressed Unconscious: Their Role in the Therapeutic Process (How the Neurosciences can Contribute to Psychoanalysis)',*International Journal Psychoanalysis*, 87(Pt 1), pp. 83–103.

Moreno, J.L. (1962) *Role Theory and Emergence of the Self*. Group Psychotherapy, Psychodrama Press.

Osborn-Greatrex, E. (2018) *1 Drama and Prison: A Study of Drama-Based Methods Used in the Aid of Rehabilitation of Offenders and the Effects on their Well-Being, Mental Health and Society*. Dissertation: The University of the West of England. https://elizabethgreatrex.com/home/drama-and-prison-a-study-of-drama-based-methods-used-in-the-aid-of-rehabilitation-of-offenders-and-the-effects-on-their-well-being-mental-health-and-society/ Accessed: 6 July 2022

Zhen-Dong, W., Baohong, C., and Qian, Z. (2020) 'The Embodiment of the Dream: Theory, Method and Technique of Embodied Imagination', *The Journal of Psychological Science*, 43(1), pp. 247–253.

# Part 2

# Education and Play Space in Dramatherapy

*Eliza Sweeney*

# 5    Learning and Therapeutic Spaces in Dramatherapy and Education

*Clive Holmwood*

This chapter will consider space in relationship to dramatherapy, its training and practice with clients and the formal and informal education of both clients and trainee dramatherapists. Space will be considered from a range of perspectives including physical, play, embodied, liminal and anthropological space, and consider practical considerations from both a dramatherapy (Jones, 1996) and educational (Holmwood, 2014), specifically an integral educational perspective (Esbjorn-Hargens *et al.*, 2010).

### Drama, Theatre, Space and Audience

In its most basic form, drama as a form of theatre has always required space. Peter Brook, in his classic publication, 'The Empty Space', states, 'I can take an empty space and call it a bare stage. A man walks across this empty space whilst someone else is watching him, and this is all that is needed for an act of theatre to be engaged' (1986, p. 11). This suggests that space is contextual, it needs a context to be placed upon it.

I have considered theatrical space in relation to the worldwide pandemic of 2020. In a book chapter (Holmwood, 2022), I developed Elam's (2001) theory that describes the idea of the 'actualization' of the dramatic world or space and compared this transformation of dramatic space to the UK government daily televised coronavirus briefings during 2020. Elam discusses two essential ingredients that make the drama: the 'situation', the place or setting, and the 'context of utterance' (2001, p. 125). I discussed that:

> The sombre wooden panels of Downing Street, the UK Government crests 'on the dais', the union jack behind the 'stay at home slogans,' and sullen tones of the speakers, could almost be mistaken for a scene from a Shakespearean tragedy; an oration of a king or prince.
>
> (Holmwood (2022: 9)

Spaces are emotionally contextual. Smith *et al.* suggest that we should pay 'geographical attention to emotion' (2009, p. 4). Other cultural geographers

DOI: 10.4324/9781003252399-8

share similar views. Tuan (2003) has considered that children, for example, respond emotionally to places in different ways to adults. Emotionally we too can respond differently to dramatic spaces. An audience member, placed in the dark of an opulent Victorian theatre, feels very different to someone sat in their front room at home, eating, drinking and talking, possibly paying little heed to the TV screen in the corner of the room. Though still an audience member of some sort, thus agreeing with Brooks idea that a theatrical space is relative in its definition by both performer and audience. I would argue this is akin to the dramatherapy space requiring a space for the therapist, client and art form. Jones describes this as the therapeutic 'triangle' (2010, p. 10). In dramatic spaces, there is then an important connection between performer, audience, space and art form.

## Dramatherapy Space

Phil Jones describes in one of his now famous nine core dramatherapy processes that 'interactive audience witnessing' (1996, p. 109) is an essential core element of dramatherapy, thus sharing parallels and similarities to theatrical space. He also suggests that 'the drama process contains the therapy' (1996, p. 4) and that the space is essential because of 'the way the therapist, the client and the art form create (the) dramatherapy space together' (2010, p. 10). There are very clear connections between dramatherapy space and theatre space as they both require some form of audience witnessing a performance or event. More importantly, it is not the space itself, but what is done in the space at a particular moment that actually defines what the space is in the 'here and now'. Hence my considerations originally in my own PhD research, later published, that dramatherapy space in schools is often 'shifting and nebulous' (2014, p. 139), as different people step into and out of the performance space often created within a dramatherapy session. Therefore, defining 'space' in which ever context, dramatic, educational or therapeutic, is not as clear as we might have at first considered. It depends upon our individual relationship to the space at a specific time and the players and audience of the space in question. We could therefore argue that space in the context of dramatherapy specifically is not only a physical space but also an embodied space as we move in it and through it with our bodies.

## Embodied Space and Play in Dramatherapy

Jones states that embodiment in dramatherapy 'concerns the way in which an individual relates to their body and develops through their body when involved in dramatic activities' (1996, p. 113). Whilst Dokter wonders 'whether the difference in human experience, as personified by cultural variables, may not influence the perception of and ability to use symbolic embodiment' (2016, p. 115). Jones therefore suggests that it is the very act of dramatic activity that allows an individual to relate to their thoughts and feelings through their body whilst Dokter suggests that this 'symbolic embodiment' is a universal manifestation regardless of cultural or social background. Embodiment is therefore universal, and our ability to access and understand our thoughts, feelings and ideas through our body is a key human endeavour. Space therefore must be defined and interpreted in relation to our embodied use of it. This is very much how Expressive Arts Therapists such as Malchiodi (2020) consider the use of the body in relation to trauma and use all of the creative arts in their work, art, dance, drama and music.

I have considered embodiment in dramatherapy before (Holmwood, 2015); more recently, I have considered embodiment in relation to neuro-dramatic play (NDP) (Holmwood, 2021a, 2022). Sue Jennings developed NDP (2011) after completing research in the Jungles of Malaysia (Jennings, 1995). I have particularly focused on one particular aspect of NDP known as embodiment, projection, role (EPR); 'a developmental play-based paradigm that can be used to assess a child's natural development, from early messy play with slime or flour and water (embodiment), to the playing with objects and beginning to make stories (projection), to fully formed characters in dramatic play and actions (role)' (Holmwood, 2021a, p. 168). Most children will have shifted through all three of these para-dynamic shifts by the time they are seven. NDP in itself is not therapy but its theoretical model is often used by many dramatherapists working with children and also at times with older adults with dementia (Holmwood, 2021b). Our own embodied internal space as well as external physical space is central to our understanding of how space is used within dramatherapy.

Again, we see that our discussion of space in dramatherapy is a complex one. It relates to personal, internal, embodied space and how this connects to the external experiences between individuals, which in itself is as I have already suggested constantly 'shifting and nebulous' (2014, p. 139); space is dependent upon the physical activity of the individuals in it and the surrounding context.

## Anthropological Cultural and Social Space in Dramatherapy

This notion of how space is constructed in therapy is not dissimilar to Jennings' observations of the use of space with the Temiar people of Malaysia, which was also an early inspiration for the development of her NDP. She observed that 'the special categories with which the Temiars conceptualize their world are off-the-ground/ground and house/forest. They regulate the human body with the upper/lower and inner/outer schemata' (1995, p. 77). Houses are built on stilts and kept above the ground. Young babies are kept in the house and not allowed to touch the ground until they are able to walk. The way the Temiar people connect with the natural space around them, including their use of ritual space in seances is intrinsically linked to their respect and understanding of nature and their cultural belief systems, which include various rituals relating to spaces around birth and death. They also believed, for example, that 'beneath the earth is a layer inhabited by demons and monsters ... (that) may cause flood waters to rise ... that inhabit river banks and river mouths' (Jennings, 1995, p. 41). That also 'the séance itself is seen as a time when the good influences in the form of small shy spirits of plants, fruits and flowers lodge on the roof of the house or the leaf decorations where the performance is taking place' (1995, p. 40). Our understanding of space is very much linked to our unique social and cultural understanding. This is exactly what Dokter was referring to earlier when she discussed the idea of 'cultural variables' (2015, p. 116) that don't impact our ability to make use of embodied symbols.

Different cultures have very different cultural understandings. In the global north, we try to keep things contained and inside. In the same way, 'lunatics', the title given to the mentally ill in Victorian England, were kept in large hospitals or asylums out in the countryside so that patients could not be seen or heard or cause distress to society (Harpin and Foster, 2014). In recent years, this westernized perspective of mental health space as being closed off, kept safe and away from society is changing. The large asylums have for the most part been closed, and care is offered in the community, though it is strongly debated as to whether all people with disabilities are truly and fully incorporated into society.

Play therapists such as Mary Chown have also advocated for play spaces to be outside and not inside (Chown, 2014). Dramatherapy spaces could therefore begin to be seen not just as physical spaces, i.e. a room, but considered in a more symbolic or metaphorical way and connected to the social, cultural and ecological understanding of each community or society.

My original work (Holmwood, 2014) considered at length the connections between drama education and dramatherapy. I was particularly interested in space from an anthropological perspective in schools when I compared drama teaching space and dramatherapy space. I described these spaces as being 'liminal'. Anthropologist Victor Turner 'describes a liminal space as being a threshold, doorway or crossing place from "limen" – a place that is neither one nor the other, a space separate or apart from the world around it' (Holmwood, 2014, p. 140). This space was defined by the context, the individual organization or school in which it occurred and the discourse or language used by the people in that institution, and that educational drama could at times be therapeutic, and dramatherapy itself could also be educational. All of this was affected through four different lenses, i.e. political, social, artistic and therapeutic (or therapy) (see Figure 5.1).

The space described was never constant, but always changing. Figure 5.1 suggests that the three outer rings are constantly moving individually but were also affected by the organization, language and art form which were also being

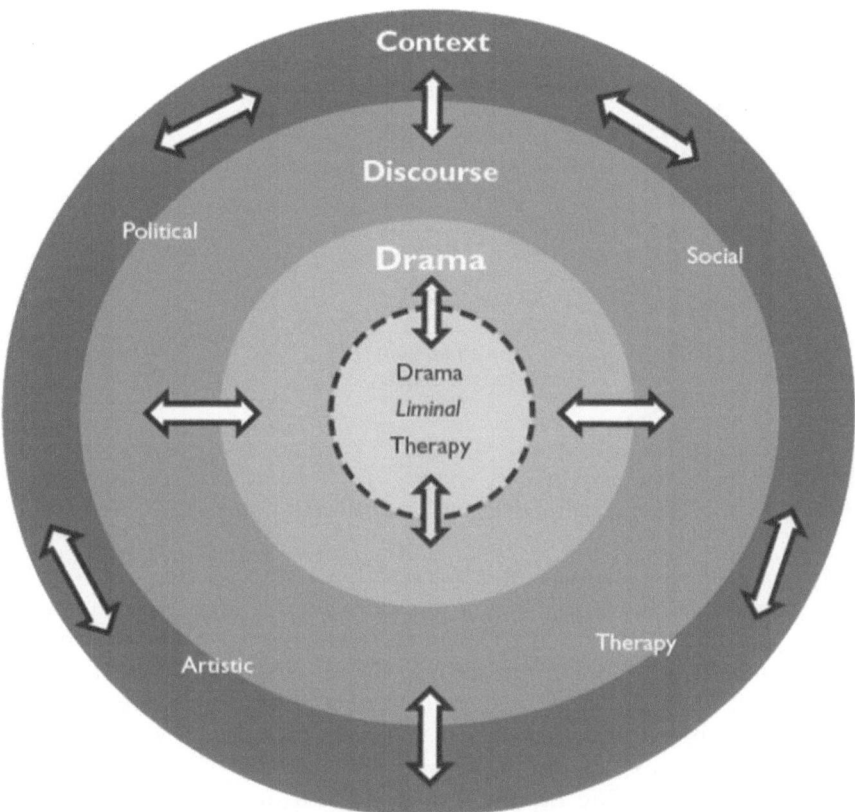

*Figure 5.1* A description of liminal dramatic and therapeutic space (Holmwood, 2014, p. 140).

pulled by the wider political, social, artistic and therapeutic concerns. At the centre of this was the drama or dramatherapy space constantly influenced by the external sources outside of it. I concluded however that this space could 'exist as a legitimate space in its own right (not as a gap between other spaces, as some might suggest) and within the wider context of the school, as the socially constructed place that surrounds the students' (2014, p. 143). Therefore, a legitimate liminal space could be formed by a group or individual, which exists in its own legitimate space, influenced by the many forces around it that pull on its shape. Like a single cell, it can then disappear as quickly when group members or individuals de-role and leave the performance space (see Figure 5.2).

I have since realized that Figure 5.1 does not really serve the complexity of these ideas as well, hence my new thinking of Figure 5.2 as a legitimate space in its own right that is elastic and can be stretched because of the influences placed upon it, but it can also change shape and even disappear instantly at the end of a dramatic activity carried out in it and return to a different form of space instantly.

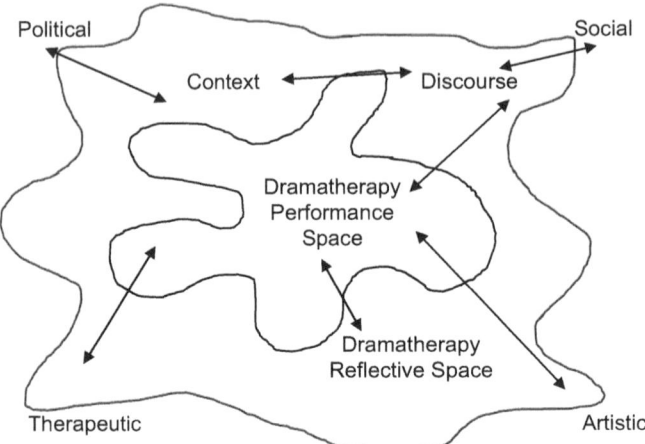

*Figure 5.2* Amorphas and elastic single-cell dramatherapy space (by C. Holmwood).

There is also the potential for a space within a space. There can be a dramatic space when individuals play a role or act out a story. Sometimes dramatherapists might use coloured material to delineate a performance space within dramatherapy. In a group setting, clients will step into this space and take on a role or act out a story and then step back out of the space at the end, whilst others observe the performance. Whether there is a physical boundary into this space or not, the moment someone steps out of or leaves the performance space, assuming no one else is still in it, it evaporates. Whilst the wider holding dramatherapy space where group members or individuals sit and reflect still exists.

### Client Spaces in Dramatherapy

If a dual amorphous dramatherapy space is reliant on client activity or reflection within it, we should also consider what actually occurs in these spaces. Clients require a regular time and safe space in which to meet. We assume that the space is confidential and in a conventional room. While talking therapies would normally require chairs, dramatherapists might require flexible, open spaces. A space in which client(s) and therapist can work creatively and dramatically and be both audience and witness to each other. Dramatherapy clients, especially those with severe learning disabilities, are often labelled as having challenging behaviour because they often struggle within the constraints of the spaces they are placed in. They are often perceived as too loud, too aggressive and too anti-social. I would argue that this has more often to do with the conventional spaces they are placed in. These spaces serve to make the lives of others around them easier, and thus become spaces these clients often feel ill at ease in.

**Vignette 1 – 'Mary'**

This notion of a conventional physical space was tested for me early in my career whilst working at a specialist day centre in the UK in the National Health Service. 'Mary' was learning disabled and nonverbal. Though she 'was an exceptional woman in her mid-thirties … Mary expressed her distress, anger and frustration by self-injurious behaviour such as banging her head on walls and floors, attempting to rip her clothes off and lashing out at those around her' (Holmwood, 2005, p. 19).

'Story' became the focus of our work together, although containing her in the actual designated therapy space was often challenging. At one stage in the therapy, we considered the story of 'The Three Little Pigs'. It contained many metaphors around space: the safety for each pig in their houses, and the differing soft to hard materials, straw, wood and brick from which each pig constructed their own house. Throughout the therapy, Mary would lead me out of the therapy room into the corridor of the small centre. Staff would come to learn that when Mary and I were together, even in the corridor, in our own performance space, they would leave us completely alone and keep a distance, whilst I told her the story of the 'Three Little Pigs'. Whilst this mobile dramatherapy space continued into the corridors of the building, I considered that 'our walls had to be strong too, not built out of straw or sticks but out of something more solid – bricks, which survive tempest more easily' (Holmwood, 2005, p. 21). However, ironically and in hindsight, I now acknowledge that this strong solid space was more elastic than rigid, as it needed to stretch around the two of us and the telling of our stories together.

What we eventually developed together was our own story about a Princess who would leave the confines of her castle and travel first to the cities, then to the towns, then the villages and the open countryside of her people, visiting them all before returning in the evenings to her castle for sumptuous parties. This act of travelling from confined to wider spaces before returning to confined spaces allowed Mary to explore the corridors of the centre and the corridors and constructed spaces of her own physical and emotional life. Though my work with her was over three years, she eventually reached a place where she was more stable and able to manage the spaces around her in her everyday life. The imaginary spaces in our stories acted as supportive structures for her to manage the actual physical spaces in her own life.

**Vignette 2 The Little Blue Man – In The Little Blue House**

Physical structures, buildings and the theme of 'home' became important containers for 'Jake' (Holmwood, 2000) who attended the same centre as Mary. Jake 'was a small slight man, who had Down's Syndrome. He had no spoken language but a wonderful sense of humour and a loud smile with accompanying voice' (2000, p. 13). Like Mary, he exhibited extreme behaviours which were difficult for himself and staff to escape from in the cramped corridors of the centre. I have expressed before that:

> Clients in Jake's position have a powerful effect on the environment and those around them. They externalise very well the inner feelings of chaos, rage and lack of A 'normal' structure to their lives, which are often not only their personal inner feelings of chaos, rage and lack of a 'normal' structure to their lives, which are often not only their personal inner feelings and early life experiences, but transversely exist in the chaotic world of the care they receive.
>
> (Holmwood, 2000, p. 14)

Jake moved from his long-term elderly carers to a home of his own shortly before he succumbed to a bout of flu and sadly passed away during the Christmas break from our work together. We were later informed by the authorities that he had been physically abused by his carers who would tie him up to manage his challenging behaviours.

Jake's physical outer world had always been chaotic, one he was never in charge of or felt safe in. Our work which was embodied and playful using soft toys and hand puppets was at first in the confines of the windowless dark sensory room full of glowing lights and colour-changing bubble tubes, perspex cylinders full of watery bubbles. We then moved to a smaller empty room, with windows and natural light, which though slightly smaller felt more open and less cramped. This move afforded us a safe physical and therapeutic space to begin to contain his experiences without the risk of any form of physical restraint. He needed a space that would contain, both his emotions and his relationships in a safe and positive way. He needed to be able to make choices for himself. He needed (sic) his own front door, which he got just before he died. I remember thinking at the time that Jake struggled his entire life to get his own space, a front door, a home that he could truly call his own. It was as if he had spent his entire life struggling for it, and once he achieved it, he no longer needed to go on. A popular song played at his funeral, one that he loved: 'you listen up here's the story about a little guy who lived in a blue world ... blue like him inside and outside, blue his house, with a blue little window ...' (Eiffel 65). For me, this song summed up Jake's life, 'he had led a very blue life' (Holmwood, 2000, p. 16).

This short vignette, like that of Mary's before, suggests that the dramatherapy space offers a containing space, one that mirrors aspects of the often-unsafe physical spaces the client's inhabit in real life, especially for those with more profound disabilities who struggle to fit into the spaces offered. The world around them expected them to fit into a utilitarian space. A constructive containing space, not only for clients' emotions but also for the relationship between client and therapist, could begin to mirror the real-world spaces they need, offering a blueprint for a safer outside world, beyond the therapy room. These supportive containing dramatherapy spaces were not constrictive but constructive, built for them and their own unique personalities, pointing to real-world possibilities. Allowing for the lack of boundary provision by others and offering them a blueprint for a possible physical and emotional space they needed in their own unique lives.

## Dramatherapy, Space and Education

An embodied physical experience allows us to understand aspects of self in new ways that can bypass our very heady, intellectual understanding of self, which can allow for new understanding and learning. In the same way, I hope Mary and Jake were able to have their own embodied physical experiences as described in the previous vignettes. The dramatherapy space allowed them to begin to find and manage the unique space each of them required in their own lives. Despite their learning disabilities and their lack of ability to speak verbally, I believe they were able to tap into this form of 'tacit' learning and learn about their own surroundings and relationship to it through the relationship with the therapist and the medium of dramatherapy. In recent years, I have also drawn parallels with this notion of embodied/knowledge and understanding from both an integral educational perspective (Esbjorn-Hargens *et al.*, 2010) and the spaces that student dramatherapists inhabit as trainees (Holmwood, 2021c), which I shall return to shortly.

There is very little disagreement with the fact that play is central to child development, education and learning. Peter Slade, one of the founding grandparents of dramatherapy (1954, 1958, 1995), and Caldwell Cook (1917) are early advocates of drama in education, both advocating for a play-based approach to education. Slade was particularly drawn to the notion of movement and shape in relation to play, which in itself requires space. However more interestingly he was the first pioneer in the UK to use the word dramatherapy and try to define the parameters of the dramatherapy space which he described as falling into three areas, '(a) conscious and intended therapy, (b) constructive education, and (c) prevention' (1958, p. 5), which he earlier described as a space 'which allows for aesthetic discovery and practice, for training of the emotions … ' (1958, p. 5). Slade was in essence trying to define these liminal spaces betwixt and between therapeutic and education, without perhaps the more sophisticated and considered language we might use today.

I shall now return to the dramatherapy space and consider it from an educational perspective and how this notion of 'education' potentially shapes an aspect of dramatherapy space from both a teacher and student perspective.

Firstly, from a teacher's perspective, I had the pleasure of delivering a practical workshop considering international approaches between drama education and dramatherapy with two American dramatherapy colleagues Andrew Gaines and Jason Butler at the Paris International Drama Education Association Conference in 2013 (Gaines *et al.*, 2015). Working with a group of almost 30 international drama educators, we considered the notion of 'aesthetic framing to more effectively and ethically serve individuals, groups or communities through drama/theatre practices' (Gaines *et al.*, 2015). We noted that many drama educators had been faced with emotional issues from their students in the context of educational drama classes, but generally felt their educational training did not equip them to manage and contain these emotional responses from students. It was noted that: 'many practitioners of applied theatre are usually quick to assert that they are not therapists, either by training or inclination and are concerned with social transformation rather than individual pathologies of rehabilitation' (Prentki and Preston, 2009, p. 12 in Gaines *et al.*, 2015). In relation to how they managed their educational teaching spaces, in the school classroom, we considered the notion of aesthetic distance, as given in Table 5.1.

*Table 5.1* Distance Model of Dramatherapy (Gaines et al., 2015; Landy, 1994)

| *Underdistance* | *Aesthetic Distance* | *Overdistance* |
| --- | --- | --- |
| Me | Me AND Not Me | Not Me |
| Reality | Liminal | Fiction |
| Impulsive | Fluid, Spontaneous | Rigid |
| Too Close | Boundaries | Withdrawn |
| Overwhelmed | Self-Regulated | Repressed |
| Manic | Grounded | Depressed |
| Fused | Related | Alienated |
| Hyper | Integrated | Dissociated |
| All | Paradox | Nothing |
| **Dramatherapy** | | |
| Dialogic oscillation modulates balance and promotes self-regulation | | |

From Gaines *et al.* (2015). Between Drama Education and Dramatherapy: International Approaches to Successful Navigation. p-e-r-f-o-r-m-a-n-c-e , 2 (1-2). http://p-e-r-f-o-r-m-a-n-c-e.org/?p=1223 (Accessed 2.5.21).

Jones (1996) also refers to the importance of this as one of his nine core processes describing it as 'empathy and distancing' (1996, p. 106). The pertinent idea being that when something in a dramatic activity is too emotionally overwhelming, or under-distanced, we move to a more distanced approach within the dramatherapy space. Story or metaphor might be used to give the client space and distance to manage the emotional issue more effectively, so that the client is not overwhelmed by the feelings. Or indeed when something is too over-distanced and the client is not connecting at all, we might adopt something less distanced such as taking on a specific role or character in order to 'walk in the shoes' of a particular character. Thus, the distance model of dramatherapy provides specific emotionally self-regulated spaces in which clients can operate safely. Empathy and distancing were also useful frameworks for both drama educators to consider 'when these overlapping realities occur outside of everyday life' (2015 np) within the context of a drama education space.

We concluded and concurred with Landy that it is within the space between the everyday and the dramatic 'that the dramatherapist best functions. His goal is to help the client better understand the everyday reality through working within the dramatic reality' (Landy, 1994, p. 26 in Gaines *et al.*, 2015). Therefore, dramatherapy spaces shift from an everyday reality to a dramatic reality, and the skilful use of empathy or distancing techniques, as appropriate, led by a dramatherapist, assists clients to negotiate these spaces safely. Allowing drama educators to gain a basic grasp of this was very helpful. We acknowledged that these dramatic realities were not exclusive to dramatherapy spaces and did and do occur within drama educational contexts too. As I previously acknowledged, drama teachers don't always feel equipped to deal with emotional issues in educational contexts. A basic understanding of how these different realities are formed within both dramatherapy and drama education settings was hopefully helpful for the drama educators present. This led to a helpful and constructive debate with the teachers present at the end of the conference session. This is something I have emphasized since in my own work (2014), that there is still much work to do in allowing drama teachers and dramatherapists to explore together both their own and their shared spaces.

The way in which space is used in the training of dramatherapists is even more complex, especially when navigating these liminal, metaphorical learning spaces connected to personal student issues and experiences. In 'The complex intersection of education and therapy in the drama therapy classroom' (2017), Butler discusses the multiple difficulties present when using practical approaches whilst training dramatherapists in Higher Education. I have already considered with my former colleague Judie Taylor (Taylor and Holmwood, 2018) that Higher Education training, in general, could be linked to a journey in itself, similar to Van Gennep's Rites of Passage (1960), with students passing through pre-liminal states on arrival at University through to post-liminal and beyond once they have graduated. Thus, liminal states exist within all educational contexts from the very beginning. However, Butler's research focused on the practicalities of how dramatherapy students are trained, using experiential pedagogy and the liminal educational/therapeutic spaces that this inhabits as part of their therapy training. Butler explains:

> Drama therapy education presents unique complexities for educators ... students engage with the techniques of their profession in order to learn how to utilize them with clients ... drama therapy is designed to work through metaphor, to subvert defences and often to indirectly arrive at client issues, it is unavoidable that students in these classrooms will have experiences that evoke their own personal affective material (2017, p. 28).

He goes on to suggest that 'This experiential learning, often accompanied by these expectations, can lead to a strong emotional response. These strong responses then lead to consequences both within and outside of the programme' (p. op cit.). In a series of interviews with trainee dramatherapists, it was acknowledged that they did at times struggle to understand the spaces which were both educational and therapeutic, but not in themselves therapy. As one student described, 'so they have like the therapy appropriate affective response, but not the therapy appropriate processing ability or space' (2017, p. 32). This further entangles and fractionalized our understanding of how educational space is used in the training of dramatherapists. The training is not in itself therapy, though students do bring personal material to the classroom space in order to reflect upon and develop their own pedagogic practice. This further enhances the complexities around how these particular spaces are used, thus agreeing with my original research in schools, that similarly in Universities these spaces can be 'shifting and nebulous' (2014, p. 139).

## Dramatherapy Space, IDBP and Integral Education

My most current thinking around this synthesis of all of these liminal spaces that I have been describing that relate to dramatherapy appears to resonate with Integral Education and in particular Integral Drama Based Pedagogy (IDBP) (Holmwood, 2021c), developed by Liwen Ma at Beijing Normal University in China. Ma's training programme has been designed for over 32 sessions for drama teachers which is an amalgam of a more emotional and embodied approach to drama, adopting integral education approaches. It is of particular interest here when considering liminal spaces and relating this to dramatherapy practice and the training of dramatherapists. Integral Education is a fusion of Indian and Chinese philosophies. Sri Aurobindo and Mirra Alfassa, known as 'The Mother' from India, and then the Confucian scholar Wang Yang Ming from China. It is broadly described as an 'emotional education' or as Ferrer et al. (2010) describe it as 'participatory [...] in which all human dimensions – body, vital, heart, mind and consciousness – are invited to co-creatively participate in the unfolding of learning and inquiry' (2010,

p. 79). This has led Ma to develop IDBP. Ma's work differs from both drama education and also dramatherapy; one could argue it is a mid-ground between the two, a form of therapeutic drama developed to assist in the training of drama educators. She suggests: 'IDBP differs from traditional educational drama courses that tend to be weak in the therapeutic function as well as differs from dramatherapy and psychological drama courses that have greater focus on healing people with serious mental health problems' (Ma and Subbiondo, 2021, p. 507).

Ma's drama teacher training considers a more embodied approach and response to the education of teachers. It also suggests that teachers should take a greater interest in the potential emotional impact that their work has on their students. It allows the teachers themselves to experience emotional embodied responses to the work from an educational perspective.

We are yet again faced with another dilemma, how might we begin to describe what occurs in such hybrid spaces such as an IDBP session, where the lines between drama education and dramatherapy blur. However, IDBP does share many of the connections discussed earlier when considering Butler's work around the training of dramatherapy students.

In relation to my previous and current thinking, I have noted that liminal spaces exist across all of these integrated, fused and amorphous professions. Within educational, therapy or dramatic contexts, there are fluid moments when something is neither therapy, education or drama. For a brief moment in that time, and in that space, it is a hybrid of all these and also none of them, which still 'exists as a legitimate space in its own right (not as a gap between other spaces, as some might suggest)' (Holmwood, 2014, p. 143). I have also considered these liminal learning spaces (Holmwood, 2019) from the perspective of a 'threshold concept', as developed by Meyer and Land, in which they state that threshold concepts: 'can be considered as akin to a portal, opening up a new and previously inaccessible ways of thinking about something. It represents a transformed way of understanding, or interpreting, or viewing something without which the learner cannot progress' (Meyer and Land, 2003, p. 1).

This 'portal' that Meyer and Land are talking about could be considered in a spatial context, not a theoretical space, but a physical space. A space in drama education, the IDBP classroom, the client lead dramathrapy space or student dramatherapy training, in which new or embodied learning of self can occur. It is only in these new legitimatized physical spaces, reached through a portal of developmental understanding, creativity, play and drama that new meanings can emerge. I am suggesting here that these spaces that are set apart from the everyday are indeed new, often temporary, but legitimate spaces in which learning and personal development can occur. To that end, the physical spaces and the creative, artistic and dramatic activities that occur within them, no matter how temporary, fulfil an exceptional and specific role in aiding each of us on our own personal therapeutic or educational journey. Without these spaces, without any of these tricky to describe, amorphous, yet legitimate, ephemeral spaces, the therapy, the education, the drama and the learning, cannot occur.

## Concluding Thoughts

This chapter has sought to consider the notion of space in relationship to drama education and dramatherapy from the perspective of the client, the therapist and the student, be they school pupils or University student training to be drama educators or dramatherapists.

All of these differing spaces and the actual roles (sic) we each play in them help to guide and shape our individual and collective relationships to these spaces. The ability to accurately describes these spaces is in fact a much more complex, difficult and nuanced task than we might at first have thought. Not only do we need to take on board the role we play, client, therapist or student, but then we need to acknowledge what we are physically doing in these spaces, how we are using and relating to our own intra-embodied experiences and how we relate this to others around us in the space. Then we need to consider the wider contexts and constraints of the organizations, regions or countries in which these physical spaces exist from a socio-cultural perspective. Finally, we need to acknowledge that spaces can appear and disappear at a moment's notice (Holmwood, 2014), depending upon the activity, dramatic act or story being told.

What I can say for certain is that these myriads of possible spaces within spaces, within spaces, are essential for our human development and growth. Our greater understanding of how each of these spaces affects and contributes to our own human therapeutic and educational development is something that I feel needs to continue for some time yet and needs further research. I am not convinced either that we will ever be completely happy with our descriptions of these spaces due to their continual amorphous nature and changing cultural perspectives. That of course doesn't mean we shouldn't try!

We have lived in very challenging times in the last few years. Covid-19 itself has made us all re-evaluate our experiences of living in separate, confined and sometimes lonely spaces for long periods of time. It is only now that we can truly begin to value the shared spaces that we inhabit together as humans; we are after all creatures who have an innate wish to want to share our space with others.

## References

Brook, P. (1986) *The Empty Space*. London: Penguin Books.

Chown, M. (2014) *Play Therapy in the Outdoors: Taking Play Therapy Out of the Playroom and into Natural Environments*. London: JKP.

Cook, C. (1917) *The Play Way*. London: William Heinmann.

Dokter, D. (2016) 'Embodiment in Dramatherapy', in Jennings, S. and Holmwood, C. (eds.) *Routledge International Handbook of Dramatherapy*. London: Routledge, pp. 115–124.

Eiffel 65 (1999) *Blue (Da Ba Dee)*. London: Warner Music UK Ltd.

Elam, K. (2001) *The Semiotics of Theatre and Drama*. 2nd Edition. London: Routledge.

Esbjorn-Hargens, S., Reams, J. and Gunnlaugson, O. (2010) *Integral Education – New Directions for Higher Learning*. New York: SUNY.

Ferrer, J. N., Romero, M. T. & Albareda, R. V. (2010). Integral transformative education: A participatory proposal. In S. Esbjo"rn-Hargens, J. Reams, & O. Gunnlaugson (Eds.), *Integral Education: New Directions for Higher Learning* (pp. 79-103).Albany, NY: SUNY Press.

Gaines, A.M., Butler, J.D. and Holmwood, C. (2015). 'Between Drama Education and Drama Therapy: International Approaches to Successful Navigation', *p-e-r-f-o-r-m-a-n-c-e*, 2 (1-2). http://p-e-r-f-o-r-m-a-n-c-e.org/?p=1223 (Accessed 2.5.21).

Harpin, A. and Foster, J. (eds.) (2014) *Performance, Madness and Psychiatry – Isolated Acts*. London: Palgrave Macmillan.

Holmwood, C. (2000) You Listen Up Here's the Story About a Little Guy Who Lived in a Blue World ... in Dramatherapy Volume: 22 issue: 3, page(s): 13-17. 10.1080/02630672.2000.9689557

Holmwood, C. (2005) 'A tale of tales', *Dramatherapy*, 27(1), pp. 19–23. DOI: 10.1080/02630672.2005.9689645

Holmwood, C. (2014) *Drama Education and Dramatherapy: Exploring the Space between Disciplines*. London: Routledge, pp. 167–177.

Holmwood, C. (2015) Dramatherapy, Tai Chi and Embodiment in Creative Arts Creative Arts in Education and Therapy, Volume 1 (2015), Issue 1, Page 63 – 75. Quotus Publishing.

Holmwood, C. (2019) 'Chapter 5: Liminality in Higher Education: Gaps and Moments of Uncertainty as Legitimate Learning Spaces', in Taylor, J. and Holmwood, C. (eds.) *Learning as a Creative and Developmental Process in Higher Education – A Therapeutic Arts Approach and Its Wider Application*. London: Routledge, pp. 61–71.

Holmwood, C. (2021a) 'Neuro-Dramatic-Play and a Hero's Journey: A Play-Based Approach in a UK Junior School', in Jennings, S. and Holmwood, C. (eds.) *Routledge International Handbook of Play, Therapeutic Play and Play Therapy*. London: Routledge.

Holmwood, C. (2021b), 'Older people, dementia and neuro-dramatic-play: A personal and theoretical drama therapy perspective', *Drama Therapy Review*, 7(1), pp. 61–75. doi: 10.1386/dtr_00061_1

Holmwood, C. (2021c) 'A Review of Drama Education (UK) and Integral Drama Based Pedagogy (China) Western and Eastern Perspectives and Influences', in *Beijing International Review of Educational*. Beijing: Brill Publishing, 3(2021), pp. 515–528.

Holmwood, C. (2022) 'Making a Story Out of a Crisis - A Response to Covid-19: A Dramatic Perspective', in Holmwood, C., Jennings, S. and Jacksties, S. (eds.) *The Routledge International Handbook of Stories and Therapeutic Storytelling*. London: Routledge, pp. 7–11.

Jennings, S. (1995) *Theatre Ritual & Transformation – The Senoi Temiars*. London: Routledge.

Jennings, S. (2011) *Healthy Attachments & Neuro-Dramatic Play*. London: JKP.

Jones, P. (1996). *Drama as Therapy, Theatre as Living*. London: Brunner Routledge.

Jones, P. (ed.) (2010). *Drama as Therapy Volume 2: Clinical Work and Research into Practice*. Hove: Routledge.

Landy, R. (1994). *Drama Therapy: Concepts, Theories, and Practices.* 2nd Edition. Springfield: Charles C. Thomas.

Ma, L. and Subbiondo, J.L. (2021) 'Integral drama based pedagogy as a practice of integral education: Facilitating', *The Journey of Personal Transformation in Beijing International Review of Education,* 3(2021), pp. 491–515.

Malchiodi, C. A. (2020).*Trauma and Expressive Arts Therapy: Brain, Body, and Imagination in the Healing Process.*The Guilford Press.

Meyer, J. and Land, R. (2003) Threshold Concepts and Troublesome Knowledge: Linkages to Ways of Thinking and Practicing Within the Disciplines. ETL Occasional Report 4. Edinburgh teaching and Learning Research Project (TLRP).

Prentki, T. and Preston, S. (2009). *The Applied Theatre Reader.* NY: Routledge.

Sladel, P. (1954) *Child Drama.* London: University of London Press.

Slade, P. (1958) *(Reprinted 2003) Dramatherapy as an Aid to Becoming a Person: Guild Lecture No 103.* London: The Guild of Pastoral Psychology.

Slade, P. (1995) *Child Play and Its Importance for Human Development.* London: JKP.

Smith, M., Davidson, J., Cameron, L. and Bondi, L. (2009) *Emotion, Place and Culture.* Farnham: Ashgate Publishing.

Taylor, J. and Holmwood, C. (eds.) (2018) *Learning as a Creative and Developmental Process in Higher Education- A Therapeutic Arts Approach and Its Wider Application.* London: Routledge.

Tuan, Y.F. (2003) *Space and Place. The Perspective of Experience.* Minneapolis: University of Minnesota Press.

Van Gennep, A. (1960) *The Rites of Passage.* London: Routledge.

# 6 Connecting Spaces
## Playing to Relate

*Sarah Mann Shaw*

## Introduction

All relationships need spaces to grow and develop, especially in children and young people whose primary relationships were experienced as abandoning and hurtful. How does a child who has learned to fear trust in relationships explore an inner vitality and accept a different relational perspective? I propose that dramatherapy, through the provision of a play space, can enable an exploration and a balancing of experience, thus supporting a different relational pattern. Trevarthen (in Hendry and Hasler, 2017: 7) writes that the newborn infant has no knowledge of facts and yet 'may imitate and synchronize with actions presented as signals for an imaginative dialogue'. Babies are born relational, and the desire to communicate and establish connections are innate strengths for social vitality. Contact with others is a primary motivating experience in human behaviour and, for the most part, it is reciprocal. Where contact is freely given, we are universally rewarded by its presence (Fairbairn, 1952; Guntrip, 1971). Without this reciprocity in relationships, an infant's sense of self and their ability to relate are significantly damaged.

This chapter will present a dramatherapy case study in which the attuned and playful presence of the dramatherapist helped to overcome a fear of trust and opened a space in which the child's inner world could be safely explored. This was developed within the play space, a space that is provided and contained by the dramatherapist and where the primary aim is to facilitate and develop play within the therapist/client relationship. In my work as a dramatherapist and child and adolescent psychotherapist with adopted children in the UK, I work with early experiences of trauma and attachment difficulties. Many of my clients have experienced a deep-seated lack of safety within their birth families, and their adoptive parents report dysregulated patterns of sleep, diet and ability to learn and relate. Adopted clients are referred to dramatherapy through the local authority supported by the Adoption Support Fund which enables adopted children and their families to access a range of therapies.

DOI: 10.4324/9781003252399-9

## Trauma

Trauma is defined as a deeply felt pervasive experience, the response to which can majorly impact a child's ability to cope with and manage relationships (Crenshaw, 2014; Perry, 2009; Schore, 2013; Siegal, 2001; Van der Kolk, 2005, 2014). It can cause feelings of helplessness and fear, diminishing a sense of self and the ability to trust that others are available to help manage distressing feelings. As a result, the defence to relationships and to the exploration of painful internal material, often held in an embodied preverbal level, is best acknowledged and responded to through a gradual process of re-engagement firstly with the self and then relationships. In dramatherapy, this process of re-engagement can be nurtured within a therapeutic play space. By creating and containing this play space, dramatherapists attend to the developmental nature of play, observing the developmental and chronological age of our clients and their relationship or non-relationship to play.

Defence mechanisms are usually defined as mental processes that operate unconsciously; they serve to regulate psychological arousal against painful emotions such as fear, terror, anxiety and loss. When a reliable other has been unavailable, we push down what has been difficult to deny it  or to forget and begin a process of isolating and excluding experiences. We push it into a place where it remains separate from ordinary integration. It remains undigested, stuck with the effect and understanding of the developmental age at which the trauma occurred (Berne, 1961; Federn, 1953; Weiss, 1950). Gammage (2017: 17) talks about the 'cloak' that enables survival in 'this imperfect relational world' and suggests that the cloak both protects and restrains our potential, stating that play has the potential to enable children to thrive. Freud wrote 'that which cannot be understood inevitably reappears; like an unlaid ghost that cannot rest until the mystery has been solved and the spell broken' (Freud, 1909: 122). As a dramatherapist, I frequently experience a child's repetition of a play theme, that will not change until some metaphorical sense has been made of the play experience and the spell has indeed been broken.

## Case Study

When working with children who have experienced traumatic disruptions to attachment, the creation of a safe space to play in the therapy room can support the validation and exploration of undigested material.

Billy, aged seven, described as being dysregulated and controlling with angry impulses, was referred to dramatherapy by the adoption support agency involved with him and his family for a dramatherapy assessment (Mann Shaw, 2016). He then went on to attend therapy with me for a year. My curiosity in working with Billy was twofold: was he able to play and how might he manage a therapeutic relationship?

Billy was removed from the care of his parents at birth due to concerns about domestic abuse and neglect. His birth mother had experienced domestic violence; she was dependent on alcohol whilst Billy was in utero and experienced depression. Four days after birth, Billy was taken to a confidential foster placement and remained with foster carers for eighteen months; these carers were later described by the social worker as *relationally inconsistent*. It is likely that the lack of a nurturing relationship from the foster carers further impacted Billy's inability to feel safe and secure and construct meaningful relationships in which he felt the presence of help, love and support in times of difficulty. I wondered how this might present itself in the therapeutic relationship and if Billy would know how to make use of me in our work together. Meares (2016) describes how the therapist creates a poetry of making relationship where previously a child has experienced attachment as disorganized. The poetry in dramatherapy is in the playful encounter of creating and inhabiting a play space with another person (Evreinov, 1927; Jennings, 2011; Jones, 2007; Slade, 1954; Winnicott, 2005). The dramatherapist can be experienced as a playful other. Do we need relationships to play or in playing do we facilitate relationships? My work with Billy suggested that it was the play space that was crucial to the evolution of a relational space in which he could tolerate, explore and enjoy being with another without creative defence.

Informed by Steve Mitchell's work on individual dramatherapy, I work with designated separate spaces. Mitchell (1995) writes about the need for a differentiation between a space in which there is an introduction and closure to the session and the space in which the creative engagement of dramatherapy takes place. My space is arranged with two sofas, for the checking-in and out phases, and an open play space.

Billy attended dramatherapy sessions with his adopted mum, Lisa. Lisa became an attuned observer to Billy's play, remaining on a sofa unless Billy invited her into the play space. During our initial parenting consultation, Lisa and I discussed how Billy might feel being observed by his mum whilst playing and how she could be invited to become a more active participant. We talked about how this may become a rhythmic dance of attachment. Lisa wondered if at times she might draw back from being a more active witness to enable Billy to have a sense of separation and autonomy in the play space whilst feeling safely engaged in the process of play. While in conversation with Lisa, I had prepared Billy a box with play objects and art materials.

---

**The Play Space: Vignette 1. The play space is ready.**

We start and end each session sitting on the sofas. Billy and Lisa sit together, and I place myself opposite them. This space offers a place for more explicit sharing of the week's events, by either Billy or Lisa, there is a clear separation of roles and a defining of boundaries between them – the family – and myself the therapist.

During the first session, Billy is shy and demonstrates a normal level of anxiety; he hangs onto Mum, but also looks beyond her at a box of play objects which are placed in a large space on the floor. I tell Billy that this open space in the room is his play space, and noticing his curiosity ask him if he would like to play. We move into the play space while Lisa stays on the sofa. In the first instance, Billy chooses cars to play with and enacts scenarios in which there are numerous crashes. After a while, Billy asks if he can add soft cushion stuffing into his box which he calls *clouds*. He places his hands into the clouds, smiles at me and tells me that it feels *good and safe*. Billy then connects the stories of the crashing cars and the clouds by placing the crashing cars into the clouds, enacting a rescue mission that leads Billy into projective play. Billy tells me that he feels *excited* by the rescue mission and that his advice to any character in the cloud who may be scared was to just *breathe in and out*.

Billy is exploring metaphors of danger, the crashing cars, and places of safety, the soft clouds, developing a connection to the play space through creating a metaphorical narrative. He played naturally, without instruction, creating a projective story world with characters using imaginative expression to express social roles, the rules of his imaginative world and his reactive feelings. In combining the two, I wondered if he was telling me something of his early and current attachment experiences, that now there was the possibility of being held in a soft place and just breathing even when difficult things happen. In a later consultation with Lisa, I learned that she had introduced breathing techniques to help Billy self-regulate. Although Billy did not initially have a safe attuned other to help him navigate difficulties successfully, his relationship with Lisa had enabled some rewiring of those initial trauma survival neurological pathways. I wondered if Billy's play would further demonstrate what his survival trauma strategies might have been and what changes had occurred because of attuned, empathic parenting in his adopted family.

### Reflections

Parten references six stages of play development (1929). Billy entered therapy at the stage of solitary play which is linked developmentally from birth to 2 years. Billy played alone and did not expect or need a fellow playmate. This was absolutely linked to the beginnings of a new relationship, with me, with his adoptive family but also with himself. At this stage of play development, an infant has not yet learned how to play with others but is capable of beginning to tell stories. Playing alone gives children the time they need to think, explore and create. When a child plays alone, they learn to concentrate, think for themselves, come up with creative ideas and regulate emotions. My role at this stage was simply to witness Billy's play. As a child and adolescent psychotherapist, I draw on Rogers' (1951) three core growth conditions: genuineness, unconditional positive regard and accurate empathy. Contact with others is a primary motivating experience in human behaviour, and meeting Billy with this relational focus enabled him to feel noticed and heard. As human beings, we need to be able to relate to our internal world, our contact with self, our sensations, feelings, fantasies, thoughts, wants and needs. When we have been traumatized by a relationship, we need to experience a reliable other who will help make sense of our pain. Billy's adoptive parents were attuned and loving therapeutic parents. The dramatherapy space supported an ability to understand trauma and facilitated a play space for Billy in which he felt neither under nor overwhelmed by his relationship to play with the dramatherapist. In play with themes of danger, he used objects in place of another character but playing with themes of safety within the clouds, his play was more sensory in nature, exploring texture and noticing how the fabric felt soft and gentle. This insight enabled him and the frightened objects in his play world to breathe gently, inducing a state of relaxation and calm. At this point in time, the relational space between myself and Billy was smaller than that of the child's imaginative world. In my role as relational witness and not as co-player, I intentionally placed my body in space to take up less of the play, offering inquiry and attunement but not too much involvement (Erskine *et al.*, 1999). My role, in this moment, was to hold the play space for Billy.

## The Play Space: Vignette 2. The Play Space Holds and Explores Danger

This is our ninth session together. Billy uses play objects to create a town located in the desert, at the mercy of the elements, and thus repeatedly threatened by tornadoes which destroy the town. Billy rebuilds the town, and the cycle starts again. The town is populated by characters who at the beginning of the play are killed by the disasters, but in this session another element is added.

Billy picks two snakes from my shelves and tells me that they are a father and his child. He tells me that they are very dangerous, and they will eat any characters they find, then manipulates the snakes to circle the town looking for people to eat. At this point, Billy introduces three more characters: one he makes play dead (freeze response), another hides (flight response) and the third prepares to fight the snakes (fight response).

### Reflections

The limbic system is sensitive to traumatic hyperarousal and is concerned with survival and instinctive trauma responses. When the limbic system perceives a threat, it releases hormones which prepare the body for defensive action. Once the traumatic event is over, cortisol halts the body's alarm system and releases different chemicals to restore a feeling of equilibrium. If a child has experienced repeated trauma, insufficient cortisol is released to stop the alarm system (Rothschild, 2000; Van der Kolk, 2014). If the limbic system perceives that there is enough time to react, then the flight response is activated. If there is not enough time but enough strength to defend, then there is a fight response, and if there is neither time nor strength, then the body will freeze. In this response state, the response time slows down, there is no fear or pain and the body is in an altered state of reality or dissociation. In Billy's story, one character lay prostrate on the floor while the snake repeatedly circled him. Billy told me that the character *'felt nothing'*. In the check-in/out space, Lisa reflected that at school and at home, Billy might be in a perpetual state of hyperarousal. We thought about how his limbic system might be continuously responding to a real or an imagined threat, thus unable to rest or relax.

Billy goes on to create a world in which the snakes remained predatory and dangerous; they kill humans using venom, letting them die and sometimes swallowing them whole, touching on themes of devoration. Billy tells me that the humans are still alive inside the snakes' bodies, *'tickling them'*. When I ask how this might be for the snake, Billy tells me that it is *'frustrating and that the snake hits itself to kill the human inside'*. This was a profound statement given that Billy's birth mum had experienced domestic violence whilst pregnant. I wondered if Billy unconsciously carried the fear of infanticide of being 'killed off' by the parent. This helped me to emphatically understand his need for control, which his parents reported as a major theme at home.

### The Play Space: Vignette 3.

From Sessions 10 to 16, Billy's imaginary world in the play space was repeatedly struck by tornadoes and tsunamis, natural environmental phenomena that had the potential to destroy everything in their path. At other times, the town was threatened by robbers, a more human threat. I wondered how the choice of these threats might symbolically represent Billy's early experience of trauma. Billy tells me that it takes *'two years for it (the town) to recover from the fires and three years to recover from the tornadoes'*. I reflect back to Billy that it takes time to recover from scary experiences. Billy goes on to say that because the townsfolk are suffering, the snakes decide to work with the Sherriff and be helpful. He explains the snakes will catch the robbers and *'vomit them'* into the Sheriff's jail. In this way, they are not internalized as bad objects but are able to be externalized and contained in a space outside of the body (from personal communications with E. Sweeney, 2021).

## Reflections

Setting up the play space each week as Billy had left it became an important part of our work together. Billy took photographs of the town space each week so that I could replicate his play space, thus offering consistency and predictability as well as an archive, a permanence that could not be forgotten. Billy would walk into the therapy room each week and after having a quick check-in, entered the play space continuing with the narrative or replicating it from the previous session while at other times developing it. It was his space, and the familiarity gave Billy a sense of ownership over his therapy. Relationally, he knew that I both held and prepared the space each week and in thus doing held him in mind. This was important play and relational space work.

Over time, Billy's play developed more complex metaphorical narratives and his play world took up more space in the room as he added characters and objects, all taking on symbolic significance. Consequently, this enabled me to take up more space in relation to both Billy and his play space: my inquiries became more frequent, my empathy for the characters and his dilemmas more pronounced. I used mentalization to try and imagine the inner world of the characters, sharing my thinking with Billy who began a dialogue with me about them and aspects of the story. Mentalization (Fongay *et al.*, 2002) is the capacity to be self-reflective and to wonder about oneself. By being curious about the character's internal experiences, I was reflecting on what it might have been like to be Billy in a frightening world, without making this explicit. In mentalizing on the characters experiences, I was utilizing aesthetic distance. Dramatherapists know that play fosters the development of an emotional language and cognition. In imagining what it might have been like to be scared, I was hoping to facilitate a link with Billy's lived experience.

## The Play Space: Vignette 4

## The Play Space Considers Safety

On arriving at his 16th dramatherapy session, Billy tells me what is going to happen in the play space, signalling that he had clearly been thinking about it in the time and space between our weekly sessions. I ask if there is anything he would like me to do. This question was to ascertain if he was ready to let me become involved in his play (thus far I had been an observer). Erskine *et al.* (1999: 85) writes that at the beginning of the therapeutic relationship, most clients are not ready for full contact. A therapy of contact in relationship 'uses the involvement of the therapist to invite the client into becoming more and more authentic, aware of himself or herself, and open to relationship'. The involvement of the therapist must consider the developmental presentation of the client, an appropriately involved therapist notices and evaluates a client's developmental age and responds to that client internally as if they were that age. Developmental appropriateness is always genuine, involves patience and is consistent with the client's presentation. In attending to this, dramatherapists can offer a play space that is developmentally connected with the inner world of the client.

Billy thinks that the townspeople should have a warning system for the tsunamis, tornadoes and any robbers which might come to town. We find some flashing orbs and a rattle, which, when sounded, indicates that the townspeople have to get into their safe place. Billy adds a play mobile fire engine with a firefighter and tells me that the firefighter has to keep a constant lookout over the town and surrounding areas and be alert to danger. He is not allowed to sleep or rest. This character's perpetual alertness supported the emergence of a more quiet and ordered play.

## Reflections

Melanie Klein (1964/1948) saw the play as a means of understanding and treating children and thought that the spontaneity of children's play was like the process of adult's free association, revealing the unconscious world to the psychoanalyst which, within the boundaries of the therapeutic relationship, allowed for interpretation. Erickson (1963) referred to play as the child's 'work', arguing that through play the child came to understand the world and his place within it. He felt that when anxiety became too great, playfulness was disrupted. In the dramatherapy play space, Billy directed his anxiety into the play. When the alarm systems sounded, the townspeople went into their safe spaces. Over the course of his play, the safe places developed from simple cardboard boxes to tents to a doll's house. We talked together about how the townspeople might feel. Through this sharing, Billy developed an emotional vocabulary for stress, anxiety, fear and safety and was perhaps able to internalize the safe space of the townspeople within his own body and psyche.

Winnicott writes that 'It is in playing and only in playing that the individual child or adult is able to be creative and to use the whole personality and it is only in being creative that the individual discovers self' (2005: 54). Winnicott's writing draws many analogies between the infant–mother/child–therapist relationship and the role of play in the relationships. He spoke of the need for the mother to establish a 'holding' or 'facilitating environment' that enabled play and development. Therapy, he goes on to say, is to do with two people playing. If the therapist cannot play, they are not suitable for the work. If the child cannot play, then something needs to be facilitated to enable this. In

Billy's case, the play space supported the development of the relational space which in turn fostered the therapeutic space.

Billy asks that I move the town people into the safe places whenever the alarm sounds, and for several sessions this was my task. He had finally invited me to play with him and designated me a role distinct from his own. We had moved into an associate play space. Associate play emerges at around the age of 3–4 years. It involves playing separately from one another but with some assistance and co-operation. Billy and I were playing next to each other but not yet working together in the play space. Billy's capacity to play and to be in a relational space with me was expanding, and yet at this stage in our work together, his play demonstrated that we were engaged in playing at an earlier developmental age than his 7 years. However, Billy had now progressed to being able to step in and out of the play and reflect on what was happening.

## Reflection

Gammage (2017) writes that this process of detaching from and reflecting on the play 'supports the later development of emotional resilience' (Gammage, 2017: 42). During this stage of our work, Billy was in charge of the destructive play in the play space. He would manipulate fabric to enact the tornadoes, demonstrating their impact on the town. His engagement with destructive play enabled him to safely express his psychological defences of fear and aggression. As Billy physicalized this element of destruction, he was aware of his own physical strength and of being in control of it. This 'displacement of meaning' (Freud, 1965; Irwin cited in Weber and Haen, 2005: 16) makes it possible for children to express frightening thoughts and feelings safely, without resistance. I started to mentalize what this constant survival from disaster might feel like for the town's people. As Nietzsche said, 'We have art so that we may not perish by the truth' (2017: 22). Billy was able to play with destruction and survival, all the while remaining spontaneous, explorative and open to the hard themes of life and of play.

My role in maintaining the survival of the townsfolk was to provide the 'holding space' (Winnicott, 1989). Billy and I had created a transitional space, holding the space between the real and imaginary world, between the 'me' and 'not me' (Winnicott, 1958: 215). Irwin (in Weber and Haen, 2005) writes that what most dramatherapists work towards are the goals of facilitating imaginative play at the highest possible level, strengthening self-control and affect regulation and helping clients put feelings and behaviours into words. After several months of work, Billy was able to communicate to his mum that dramatherapy helped him feel '*less sad*'.

### The Play Space. Vignette 5.

### The Play Space Explores the Body

It is session 28. Looking at my play objects, Billy asks for the play heart and brain from my shelves. Using these and beach shells, he constructs a body in the middle of the play space. Billy gives the body two brains, one large and one small, and adds arms, legs and a tummy. He also gives the body a memory. The memory has two parts, an upper memory for those memories that can be remembered and a lower part for the older memories that cannot always be remembered but are still there. He fills both parts of the brain with buttons. I talk about how the body holds memory and how when we are very young, we don't have clear memories but that these earlier memories are held differently within the body. Billy listens and decides to keep the door to both parts of the memory open. Billy places some of the buttons from the lower part in a shell representing the body's tummy. I was struck by Billy's under-standing and representation of trauma and memory in the body and the play space. At this moment, the play space and the body are united. He then asks if we can draw together. At first, we make marks with pastels, smearing colours and textures over paper, gestures that feel develop-mentally young for his age, but Billy takes delight in smudging and creating messy work, and I take delight in his. Over the next few sessions, the pictures became more structured, taking form. Billy tells me he '*is a genius*', that his work is '*so good*', proudly showing his mum.

Returning to the play world in the following sessions, Billy and I continue to play with themes of danger and safety. In thinking about how the characters in these worlds manage, Billy tells me that 'they *are all safe and rested now, there's a bubble over and around the town keeping it safe*'. Billy says of these newly constructed worlds, '*if it falls down, we can build it together again*'. I wonder if this was perhaps an expression of the merging of the play and the relational spaces. In this statement, Billy demonstrated that he had reached the developmental stage of co-operative play, in which there is a sharing of the play space and a playful relationship with other. The play space had become more expansive, the relational contact between Billy and I had become useful to him and Billy had psychologically grown. Billy had strengthened his internal space through the play with the external space and worlds created. I hoped that in the next moment of crisis or fear that Billy would be able to build themself back up again, like the worlds in the play space, with the traumatic sensations having been replaced with something more resilient and structurally sound.

## Conclusion

Earlier in this chapter, I posed the question, 'Can a child, who has learned to fear trust in relationships, explore an inner vitality and accept a different relational perspective'?

The creation of a holding play space in dramatherapy creates a potential space for exploration, which Winnicott referred to as a transitional space, a place of change, growth and coming into oneself (Winnicott, 2005). Billy had learned to fear relationships and, as a result, had constructed creative defences of self-sufficiency and control within himself. In this way, he did not have to risk encounter with another. Relational therapy carried a risk of contact. From the first session, Billy's gaze was drawn to the play space and the box of play objects that I had initially prepared for him.

Billy was instinctively and naturally drawn to play, and as presented in this chapter, Billy's dramatherapy had journeyed through Parten's six stages of play development (1929). At home, Billy could play at the parallel play stage; he played alongside 'other', and any attempt the family made to include Billy in associate or collaborative play became competitive. Billy could not accept the play position of the other at home, whereas in dramatherapy, when we came to these stages of play, this was markedly different.

Over the course of our year together, Billy's play developed from using symbols and simple narratives to complex metaphorical narratives with characters. His language developed from being purely descriptive to being able to imagine what the themes in his created world might mean for the characters within it. He utilized the 'healing effect of the dramatic "as if"' (Duggan and Grainger, 1997: 99). Billy, in imagining the character's plight, was able to think and feel as if someone else, paradoxically making meaning of his internal world. Billy developed an emotional narrative. As his preoccupation with disaster abated, he was able to pronounce himself as a 'genius', taking true delight in his successes in play and marking a rise in self-esteem. These were significant developments.

Equally significant was the development in the play relationship between Billy and myself. Initially, Billy was a solo player, and I witnessed his play and gently reflected this back to him. I was in the play space and alongside him but remained at a relational distance to his play, allowing him space to discover and create. As Billy's play developed and themes and metaphors became expanded upon, I moved relationally closer to the play using Roger's core conditions. I demonstrated interest and inquiry in the stories, the characters, his world and the dilemmas presented. I wondered what he felt about his world and accepted and normalized Billy's responses. In moving into associate play, I was invited to move closer to the play space and given a role to play. Billy created the destructive element of the play, and I was designated the role of maintaining safety for the characters. In knowing that his characters would not be harmed, Billy was able to fully embody more destructive elements. For a while, each session followed a cycle of destruction and regeneration. The dangers became more extreme and the chance of survival more fragile, and yet the characters did survive, just as Billy had. The associate play stage enabled a core element to be held by the therapist supporting Billy to explore destruction with less vulnerability. Finally, we moved to co-operative play, a stage of play that usually emerges at four years or more. In this play, I took more play risks, whilst remaining attuned to Billy and his responses. We played games that involved winning and losing which Billy not only managed well but took delight in our collaborative efforts. We taught and learned from each other. The play became more spontaneous; it was imaginative and active, and I could contribute more which also made Billy laugh. Our play became more sociable whilst still remaining controlled and directed by Billy.

Play is relational and we attend to it with an attuned awareness of those we invite into it. We carefully consider our clients' capacity for contact; we listen, observe, express empathy, make inquiries and are prepared to play, for it is in the connection of the two that a child can re-engage with an inner sense of vitality that is fundamental to their lived experience.

## References

Berne, E. (1961) *Transactional Analysis in Psychotherapy: A Systemic Individual and Social Psychiatry*. New York: Grove Press.

Crenshaw, D. (2014) 'Play Therapy Approaches to Attachment Issues', in Malchiodi, C. and Crenshaw, D. (eds.) *Creative Arts and Play Therapy for Attachment Problems*. Guildford Press.

Duggan, M. and Grainger, R. (1997) *Imagination, Identification and Catharsis in Theatre and Therapy*. London: Jessica Kingsley Publishers.

Erickson, E. (1963) *Child and Society*. 2nd ed. New York: W.W. Norton.

Erskine, R., Moursund, J. and Trautman, R. (1999) *Beyond Empathy. A Theory of Contact in Relationship*. Philadelphia and London: Brunner Mazel.

Evreinov, N. (1927) *The Theatre in Life*. New York: Harrap.

Fairbairn, W.R.D. (1952) *An Objects Relation Theory of Personality*. New York: Basic Books.

Federn, P. (1953/1977) *Ego, Personality, and the Psychoses*. London: Maresfield Reprint (original work published 1953).

Fongay, P., Gergely, G., Jurist, E.L. and Target, M. (2002) *Affect Regulation, Mentalization and the Development of the Self*. New York: Other Press.

Freud, A. (1965) *Normality and Pathology in Childhood: Assessments of Development*. 92nd ed. New York: International Universities Press.

Freud, S. (1909). *Collected Papers* (Vol. 3). London: Hogarth.

Gammage, D. (2017) *Playful Awakening Releasing the Gift of Play in Your Life*. London: Jessica Kingsley Publishers.

Guntrip, H.J.S. (1971) *Psychoanalytic Theory, Therapy and the Self*. New York: Basic Books.

Irwin, E. (2005) 'Facilitating Play with Non-Players', in Weber, A.M. and Haen, C. (eds.) *Clinical Applications of Drama Therapy in Child and Adolescent Treatment*. New York and Dove: Brunner Routledge.

Jennings, S. (2011) *Healthy Attachments and Neuro-Dramatic Play.* London: Jessica Kingsley Publishers.

Jones, P. (2007) *Drama as Therapy, Theory, Practice, and Research.* London and New York: Routledge.

Klein, M. (1964) *Contributions to Psychoanalysis 1921–1945: Developments in Child and Adolescent Psychology.* New York: McGraw-Hill (Original work published 1948).

Mann Shaw, S. (2016) 'Stevie and the Little Dinosaur: A Story of Assessment in Dramatherapy', in Jennings, S. and Holmwood, C. (eds.) *Routledge International Handbook of Dramatherapy.* Oxon: Routledge.

Meares, R. (2016) *The Poets Voice in the Making of the Mind.* London/New York: Routledge.

Mitchell, S. (1995) *Clinical Studies in Dramatherapy.* London: Jessica Kingsley Publishers.

Nietzsche, F. (2017) *Translated by Hill R.K. and Scarpitti M.A. A Will to Power.* London: Penguin Classics.

Perry, B. (2009) 'Examining child maltreatment through a neurodevelopmental lens: Clinical application of the neurosequential model of therapeutics', *Journal of Loss and Trauma,* 14, pp. 240–255.

Rogers, C. (1951) *Client Centred Therapy.* Boston: Houghton Mifflin.

Rothschild, B. (2000) *The Body Remembers. The Psychophysiology of Trauma and Trauma Treatments.* New York: V.W. Norton.

Schore, A. (2013) 'Relational Trauma, Brain Development and Dissociation', in Ford, J. and Courtois, C. (eds.) *Treating Complex Traumatic Stress Disorder in Children and Adolescents.* New York: Guildford Press.

Siegal, D. (2001) 'Towards an interpersonal neurobiology of the developing mind: Attachment relationships, 'mindsight', and neural integration', *Infant Mental Health Journal,* 22(1–2), pp. 67–94.

Slade, P. (1954) *Child Drama.* London: University Press.

Trevarthen, C. (2017) 'Foreword', in Hendry, A. and Hasler, J. (eds.) *Creative Therapies for Complex Trauma.* London and Philadelphia: Jessica Kingsley Publishers, pp. 7–9.

Van der Kolk, B. (2005) 'Developmental trauma disorder: A new rational diagnosis for children with complex trauma disorders', *Psychiatric Annals,* 35(5), pp. 401–408.

Van der Kolk, B. (2014) *The Body Keeps the Score: Brain, Mind Body in the Healing of Trauma.* New York: Viking.

Weiss, E. (1950) *Principles of Psychodynamics.* New York: Grune and Stratton.

Winnicott, D.W. (1958) Collected Papers: Through Paediatrics to Psycho-Analysis by D. W. Winnicott (1958-12-01) London Tavistock Publications Ltd.

Winnicott, D.W. (1989) *Psychoanalytic Explorations.* Boston: Harvard University Press.

Winnicott, D.W. (2005) *Playing and Reality.* London: Routledge Classic.

# 7 Essential Factors Both Practical and Imaginal for Defining the Dramatherapy Play Space in Special Education

*Amanda Musicka-Williams*

This chapter reflects on the pivotal role that relationship to 'space' plays within dramatherapy conducted in special education. Drawing on reflections from research and long-term practice in special education, I present for discussion essential factors that have assisted the co-creation and maintenance of a dramatherapy space relevant to participants' therapeutic needs and the overall aims of the educational context. This discussion focuses on four key constructions of space which relate to the creation of a dramatherapy space in special education. These four are as follows: psychological space, physical space, imaginal space and intersubjective or relational space. They represent four conceptualizations of space that I, as a dramatherapist, consistently engage with when facilitating dramatherapy which caters to the individualized needs of a special education community.

Discussion of the first conceptualization of space, the psychological space, focuses upon environmental and cultural variables which influence the maintenance of a healthy psychological space for young participants, who due to diverse means of self-expression experience limited opportunity for voice and agency. In reflecting on the physical conceptualization of space, practical ways to create and preserve a dramatherapy space in a school, where the emphasis is on learning rather than a therapeutic process, are presented and discussed. In exploring imaginal space as a constructed reality, essential dramatic tools and methods which support young people in special education to consciously enter and exit dramatic reality are identified. In concluding these reflections on essential elements defining an accessible and inclusive dramatherapy space, I reflect overall on how we co-create and sustain an interdependent, relational space which enables a meaningful therapeutic experience for young people with disabilities. Throughout the chapter, practice and research vignettes illustrate participants' engagement with space in its multiple forms. In exploring different conceptualizations of space and the related essential factors that assist its construction, I present an argument for why space and participants' multifaceted relationship to it are pivotal to enabling the unique experience that dramatherapy offers young people in special education.

DOI: 10.4324/9781003252399-10

## Introduction

Space is both an abstract concept and a lived experience. Every day we engage with space in one form or another. Our relationship to the spaces we inhabit and what we encounter there greatly influence the quality of our daily experiences. Whether public or communal spaces, private home environments, educational settings or places of specific practice that effect recognition of commonalities and communal belonging, how we relate to everyday spaces has a significant impact on an individual's sense of self and well-being (Curtis, 2016).

In dramatherapy, we recognize multiple influences which impact partici-pant's therapeutic experience (Cassidy *et al.,* 2014, 2017; Jones, 2016). Creative engagement with space is recognized as fundamental to dramatic practice. Characteristics of space and participants' engagement with it influence both dramatherapy facilitation and how participants respond. As dramathera-pists, we invite participants to reconstruct space in ways which illuminate un-derlying therapeutic possibilities within the theatrical experience, possibilities which may be bridged into real-life encounters. We offer a therapeutic blurring of the lines between real and imagined spaces, a practice which we refer to as engaging with 'dramatic reality' (Pendzik, 2006). In dramatizations, we play with intersubjective space in ways which enable participants to redefine who they are in relationship to the world and others (Pitruzzella, 2017). In these transformative processes, engagement with space is fundamental. The dra-matherapy 'play space' constitutes a liminal, in-between space that bridges participants in playful ways, towards new experience (Johnson, 2009). There is something magical about the dramatherapy space and there is also something very real and concrete about engaging with possibility through dramatic play. Dramatherapy enables a rehearsal space for real-life encounters in ways which are accessible and developmentally appropriate for young people with intel-lectual/developmental disabilities (Bailey, 2010).

As a long-term practitioner of dramatherapy in special education, I am consistently reminded of the profound impact on therapeutic practice that 'space' has. I am also reminded of the unique ways in which individuals en-gage with space in its various forms, physical, psychological, relational and imaginal. It reminds me of how our relationship to space and subsequent engagement with it is informed by our unique experiences and ways of inter-relating. By tuning into the possibilities of 'space' in dramatherapy conducted in special education, young people with diverse ways of being are offered opportunities to explore extended experiences of themselves in ways which enhance therapeutic outcomes.

## Defining Essential Features of the Dramatherapy Space in Special Education

I define here, four essential conceptualizations of space which inform a co-created dramatherapy experience that enables and honours the diversity present within special education.

1  Psychological space
2  Physical space
3  Imaginal space
4  Intersubjective/Relational space

Practice vignettes included throughout this chapter illustrate some of the concepts explored and include reference to participant reflections from practitioner-based research. Participant names are changed to preserve anonymity, whilst responses in their own words are illustrated by italics.

### Psychological Space

Presentation of the first conceptualization of space recognizes the need to construct and manage the dramatherapy space in practical ways which promote a healthy psychological space that encourages creativity and therapeutic experience. In the context of special education, I define a healthy psychological space as one which promotes trust in the therapeutic relationship and dramatic art form, enabling participants room to grow, express themselves and their capacity for creative innovation. Construction of a dramatherapy space that meets these objectives needs to consider specific environmental and cultural variables which influence the maintenance of a healthy psychological space for young participants, who, due to diverse means of self-expression, experience limited opportunity for voice and agency.

Research exploring potential factors which enhance the mental health and self-image of young people with intellectual/developmental disabilities indicates that social connectedness has a major impact on overall well-being (Gaspar *et al.*, 2016). There is also recognition that opportunities to socially engage are limited by environments and practices which are not constructed for people with disabilities (Allan, 2014; Ineland and Sauer, 2016). Communal environments challenge young people with disabilities through their inaccessibility and by inadequately reflecting or engaging with unique disability cultures (Goodley *et al.*, 2016).

Recognizing that participants entering dramatherapy from within a special educational context have their own unique ways of engaging with both physical and relational space, there is a need to construct a space which promotes psychological safety through the permission it offers participants to create and present as their authentic selves. In order for participants to bring their authentic selves to therapy, they need to feel they are in a safe space, accompanied by a safe companion. Whilst there are significant challenges in responding effectively to the diverse self-presentations in special education, there exist practical ways to co-create a dramatherapy space, which enables psychological safety.

### The 'Save Them' Space

The following vignette explores one young boy's response to the gradual introduction of a play-based conceptualization of 'safe space'. It aims to demonstrate what's possible when the dramatherapy space promotes psychological safety in a way that is both tangible and palatable for a young person with a moderate intellectual disability and significant early life trauma.

Joe was seven when he began attending dramatherapy. He had experienced significant early life abuse and neglect. This presented as reactive distrust in others and challenging behaviours which were impulsive and often dangerous. However, Joe was resilient and creative. He liked to play with toys, directing dramatic narratives. The goal in dramatherapy was to enable Joe a contained expression of lived experiences, whilst encouraging him to explore new possibilities for relating to others. His play was challenging and repetitive. He defaulted to violent narratives in which the toys were abused. I understood that this represented his own experiences, and sometimes he reflected on this himself by talking directly about his familial experiences and offering raw emotional responses. I felt as the therapist that I needed to propose a different experience, a new narrative space, lest he become stuck in an endless replay of abuse.

I invited Joe to explore the idea of a safe space by constructing one in the room. I used a sign and some toy fencing. I explained that the toys should have a choice, somewhere safe to go where they wouldn't get hurt if they desired. Initially, Joe dismantled this space. Persisting, I re-built it. I understood that Joe's experiences had not enabled him any internalized understanding of what a safe space was or would feel like. I hoped that in concretizing the concept and inviting him to play in it, a beginning understanding of the possibilities inherent in a safe space could begin to grow.

After a period of dismantling the safe space, Joe and the toys played around it. The presence of the space at this time was becoming tolerable. The next shift occurred sometime later when, upon entering the room, Joe instructed me to set up the safe space, and over time he began to help. I witnessed his willingness to engage with the idea of this safe space growing.

A major shift happened one session when Joe placed the toys in my hand and asked me to '*save them*', whilst nodding towards the space. From that encounter on, there were always some toys that made it to the safe space. Eventually, Joe took them there himself. From this safe space and using his rescued toys as memory objects, Joe began to talk more about the experiences and feelings that each toy represented. This process occurred over many years in therapy together. The trauma of Joe's early life experiences coupled with his intellectual capacity meant that consistency, repetition and ultimately perseverance in the dramatherapy process were needed to create a 'safe enough space'. Recalling time with Joe, I often wondered whether it was the concrete creation of safe space or our ability to tolerate together the not-safe space that invited a new experience; Joe's potential to hold psychological space for both safe and unsafe experiences in creative co-existence.

*Private Space*

Establishing and maintaining a dramatherapy space in special education presents the dramatherapist with challenges. Teaching and support staff need to be educated about therapeutic process, dramatherapy practice and its potential benefits for student well-being (Holmwood, 2014; Roger, 2012). Students in special education need to be enabled, and often physically supported, to attend dramatherapy. A therapy friendly culture needs to develop which ensures development and preservation of the therapeutic space (Roger, 2012). From that basis, trust in the dramatherapy space and process can also be established with participants.

Trust in the therapeutic process is supported by the necessary safety and containment which accompany the experience of therapy as a private space. School environments offer many disruptions to privacy. In special education, this is complicated by students' need for support in daily living tasks. This level of dependence often results in limited experiences of personal privacy. The dramatherapy space gives an important opportunity for participants to experience a private space, a space where they can choose how, when and what they want to share of themselves. It is a private space which offers accessible and creative mediums for authentic self-expression and affords participants important opportunities for choice and agency.

*Ritualized Play Space*

Consistency and repetition are important in therapeutic work. In dramatherapy, we acknowledge this via our tendency to play with ritualized processes for meaning-making (Mussa, 2016; Smail, 2013). In special education, where participants require extended repetition and processing time to integrate new experiences, ritualized processes are fundamental to the construction of a safe space and group culture (Crimmens, 2006). Repetitive play rituals at the beginning and ending of sessions define the dramatherapy space and experience through consistency and containment (Mussa, 2016). With many participants in special education exhibiting ritualized behaviour, engagement in pattern-making through movement and sound invites connection and comfort through familiarity of expression. Rituals initiated and led by the young people offer opportunity for agency and a sense of ownership over the dramatherapy space and experience.

## The 'Come Find Me' Space

The following vignette illustrates an important and commonly expressed hide and seek ritual. In sharing this vignette, I aim to illustrate how participants in special education claim ownership of both private space and ritualized practice by dramatically redefining the play space to meet self-directed therapeutic objectives.

'*I am hiding and you don't know where I am*'. Henry begins every session with this script. He is 11, has a diagnosis of mild intellectual disability and autism spectrum disorder and a complex early history. Henry has accessed dramatherapy for several years, his engagement shifting from repetitive construction of play monuments in patterned formations across the space to performing dramatic narratives with puppets. Henry is self-directed and displays limited tolerance for dramatic offers from others. His invitation to '*Come and find me*' is reminiscent of Winnicott's theory that, whilst it's a joy to hide, it's a disaster not to be found (1971). I respond to his invitation by deliberately not finding him straight away, because, as Winnicott pointed out, joy resides in the 'anticipation' of being found (1971). In directing a ritualized space and process, Henry is able to trust he will 'eventually' be found. He hides in the same place and I search: '*Are you in the toy box? ... No ... Are you in the dollhouse? ... No ... Are you in the costumes? ... No ... You must be in the puppet theatre?*' I pull back the curtains, revealing a magnanimous grin, sometimes accompanied by a '*Boo*', to which I respond with melodramatic fright. Henry's grin widens. The puppet theatre doubles as his cubby house, a safe house and the space he returns to throughout the session. From this space, he enables himself to be both witnessed through the projective device of puppetry and to maintain some sense of invisibility as he narrates his experiences through the distanced perspective of a character. Occasionally I am invited in. In these moments, we are ourselves and the play is a direct interaction between us, within the imagined space of a new home. He tells me, '*It's good to have your own space*'.

## Physical Space

In discussing the second essential conceptualization of space relevant to creating a dramatherapy space in special education, practical considerations related to how the physical environment influences and enables participants' active engagement in dramatherapy are presented. These include consideration of the therapy space's location, size and accessibility. The inclusion of material objects and how they influence or define the therapeutic space and process are also discussed. Reflections on these practical elements of space invite detailed consideration of how the materiality of the dramatherapy space serves to enhance or inhibit therapeutic outcomes for participants with diverse self-presentations, capabilities and preferences.

### A 'Good Enough' Therapy Space

Communal spaces readily inhabited by others are often constructed in ways which are inaccessible to young people with disabilities (Anaby *et al.*, 2013). The dramatherapy space needs to be established in ways that enable young disabled people to engage with it, as actors and agents of their own therapeutic experience (Booker, 2011). There is a current emphasis in education and wider contexts on young people's voice and agency (Jones, 2009; Jones and Elmer, 2019). This presents unique challenges in special education, as opportunities for input afforded to other students often prove inaccessible to those with intellectual/developmental disabilities. The dramatherapy space needs to be constructed in ways which avoid perpetuating disabling experiences. Multiple elements of the physical space require management.

Not every school offers a designated therapeutic space, and flexibility in practice is vital within the special educational context. Participants often express difficulty transferring between different settings. In these cases, the work of the dramatherapist constitutes a spontaneous response within an immediate environment. Whilst Winnicott refers to the 'good enough mother' as a containing experience in therapeutic practice (1971), I will refer to the 'good enough therapeutic space' as one which is constructed to address the immediacy of participant's needs. A 'good enough' therapeutic space requires concrete markers to define the therapeutic experience. In special education, this may be provided by engaging participant's dominant senses, where others may be absent or impaired, engaging with ritualized practices which address the participant's unique preferences/modes of expression, and through the inclusion of familiar props. Often, associations with space and practice are created through visual or tactile input; however, depending on the young person's self-presentation, sounds and/or sense of smell can also be evocative tools. In constructing dramatic scenarios, a sensory-based establishment of theatrical *mis-en-scene* effectively cues participants into the fact that dramatherapy is about to occur (Booker, 2011). A 'good enough' therapeutic space can be spontaneously created in a way that enables consistency of experience without a designated therapeutic space.

In one school where I have undertaken long-term practice, dramatherapy has its own space. Participants refer to it as *'the playroom'*. A small intimate space contrasts with their classroom and has provided containment for those who present with challenging behaviours or become easily overwhelmed by new experiences. In catering to participants' unique expressions, the dramatherapy space manages a balance between offering enough space for free movement and play, whilst also promoting the relational intimacy that is fundamental to a therapeutic experience. Preparing a designated dramatherapy space for sessional work in special education involves constructing the space in a way that enables continuity between sessions. Fundamental elements of the space need to look and feel the same for participants from week to week. The space and objects within it are reconstructed to suit different participants and therapeutic objectives. The choice of what needs to stay within and what needs to go from the space is directed by participant's responses. This provides another means by which to acknowledge in a practical way participant's voice and agency, as participants effectively make choices about what informs and impacts their dramatherapy experience.

Contrasting examples of the ways in which the space is set up to meet the differing needs of participants in special education are briefly described in Table 7.1. These notes give instructions for changes that need to happen between sessions and offer examples of the practical ways in which I reconstruct the dramatherapy space to enhance the individual process.

*Table 7.1* Contrasting Examples of the Ways in Which the Space Is Set Up to Meet Differing Needs of Participants in Special Education

| Participant | Space Preparations |
| --- | --- |
| Molly (early years) New student, shy/reluctant to engage, hearing impaired, Down Syndrome, beginning to play with embodied mirroring. | Mat in centre of the room to define the movement/mirroring space. Textured ball in the centre of the mat as consistent check-in object. Room stripped of unnecessary play items to encourage focus. Transportable puppet theatre in back corner for Molly's break space. Limited fabrics in opposing corner. Avoid over stimulus, and provide limited sensory experiences through play items. |
| Peter (senior school) Moderate intellectual disability. Final year of school. Exploring emerging adult identity. | Peter's therapeutic alliance, in the form of mutually agreed upon rules, is displayed on the wall alongside his artwork as requested. In the room, there is no mat, senior chairs and conversation cards in the centre of the room as consistent check-in prompt, art materials, accessible for story-making, sand tray and other items at hand for projective work. The puppet theatre, dollhouse and early years play items removed. |
| Group work – (Middle school) Personal development programme; focused on developing respectful relationships. | Mat and drum in the centre as consistent group check-in item. Feelings poster and group rules on wall. Matching feeling cards for check-in. Limited play objects in room related to body/co-operative play each week. Unnecessary items stored away to avoid distraction. |

The dramatherapy space should be inviting. In special education, the use of objects, materials and dramatic props has played a pivotal role in engaging participants in dramatherapy (Crimmens, 2006). Recognition is given to participant's diverse preferences and intolerances when deciding what to include. Too much stimulus is overwhelming for participants with specific sensory needs, whilst not enough of the right kind of materials can result in disengagement. Inclusion of play materials offering different kinds of sensory input, such as sand trays, modelling clay, different textured fabrics, paper and cardboard that can be torn and reconstructed, sensory toys, musical instruments and other items offering sensorial and/or cause and effect experiences, is paramount to meeting the play needs of participants representing a wide range of developmental stages (Jennings, 2011).

### Imaginative Space

Dramatherapy provides an invitation into an imaginal space where all possibilities are invited for the playing (Johnson, 2009) including new roles, ways of being, interacting and experiencing (Sajnani, 2016). 'By functioning in the *as if* participants start reverberations that transcend life circumstances, generating a sense of competence and agency' (Dunne, 2009: 176). This potential to experience newness offers something particularly valuable to young people in special education. Dramatherapy offers a potential space for self-advocacy, where limiting perceptions about what it is to be a young person living with an intellectual/developmental disability can be challenged: 'in dramatherapy, you can try something new, be something different. Because we are all of us, lots of things' (Musicka-Williams, 2020a, 2020b). Inviting young people with intellectual/developmental disabilities into the imaginative space requires a scaffolded approach relevant to participant's abilities (Chesner, 1995; Crimmens, 2006). It's been proposed that people with intellectual disabilities demonstrate a tendency to be more concrete in dramatic enactments, preferring to act out scenarios which resemble real life (Bailey, 2010). In my own practice, I have encountered this. However, I have also encountered the opposite, where participants express an imaginative capacity and readiness to play that are beyond what occurs in other settings. Participants who immerse themselves in the dramatic experience can then demonstrate a reluctance or inability to leave elements of the imaginal space behind. In these moments, the physical space of the dramatherapy room becomes an important grounding point. In the following section, I explore how the imaginal space needs to be concretely constructed and deconstructed with participants in special education to enable safe passage between dramatic reality and one's potential and recognition of the here and now.

### Imitation as a Bridging Space

For participants who struggle to spontaneously engage with imaginative play, providing a bridge into dramatic action is pivotal to enabling imaginal possibilities (Musicka-Williams, 2020a, 2020b). Dramatic imitation or as participants themselves call it *'copying others'* is one method that consistently enables young participants in special education to engage in dramatic play. Physical and dramatic imitation of others provides a transitional space between self and other. By imitating others, participants begin to explore an extension of self without the pressure to be spontaneous (Musicka-Williams, 2020a, 2020b). The following vignettes, taken from recent research with adolescents in special education who explored their relationships with others through group dramatherapy, illustrate the use of dramatic imitation as a pathway to a new experience of self Musicka-Williams, 2020a, 2020b).

### I Copy the Others

Hyber participated in group dramatherapy and chose a pseudonym she felt reflected her personality. Hyber was 17 and soon to be a graduate. She loved all creative activities, particularly performing onstage. Whilst exuberantly social, Hyber didn't always receive the desired response from peers. She explained:

> *'I feel sad and left out when I just want to be included ... In dramatherapy it's different. In dramatherapy there's lots of copying and copying is good. I copy the others and then I know what to do, how to behave, how to be ... I am included. It's good. I wish there was more copying elsewhere'.*
>
> (Musicka-Williams, 2020a)

Hyber found entrance into new roles by dramatically imitating the self-presentations of others (Fischer, 2016; Landy, 1993; Musicka-Williams, 2020b). By copying peers in dramatherapy, Hyber connected to the adolescent tribe, creating inside herself a space for a new role. Imitation served as an embodied bridging space between herself and the others where she could enact the group's expected behaviours in ways which invited inclusion, successfully transferring an imagined reality into a real-world space. In response, the group not only included her more but through dramatic play they also offered her a longed-for opportunity to occasionally lead the peer tendency to imitate one another when they accepted, adopted and embodied some of her own dramatic ideas about youth roles, experiences and encounters.

### Defining Imaginal Space

Understanding the difference between the real and the imagined can be confusing for people with intellectual disability. In special education, concrete markers may be needed to distinguish between dramatic experience and return to everyday reality. This delineation needs to be comprehended before participants can begin to reflect on and integrate (at whatever capacity by which they are able to do so) what they can transfer from dramatic encounter to real life. Ways in which the dramatherapist might actively seek to illustrate a clear entrance and exit from the dramatherapy space and imaginal world for participants include opening and closing rituals (Smail, 2013) such as imaginary/gestural representation of parting the theatrical curtain, opening and closing the storybook or physically journeying to the scenic scape of the dramatic encounter. Similarly, props can be used to redefine a classroom space and cue participants into the idea of engaging with dramatic reality and their own potential.

### Co-Creating Imaginal Space

The following reflections are reconstructed from research data. These reflections present a process for consciously enacting and deconstructing the dramatherapy space alongside participants in special education. During the research project, group participants actively engaged in the reconceptualization of space. Consistent signage was used to distinguish dramatherapy from other classroom experiences. An introduction of simple, consistent props and the reconfiguration of furniture and bodies in the space communicated this change.

*'So, you're here to mess up our classroom again?'* one of the participants teases on my entrance into their classroom for our weekly dramatherapy session.

*'Yep. Sorry about that. Are you going to help me make the space? I promise we will put it back together again after'.* Participants groaned or laughed, stepping in to help redefine the space.

Participants hung a sign on the door signifying to others that the space was now designated for dramatherapy and wasn't to be disturbed. They indicated the 'performing space' – where dramatic enactments were rehearsed and shared – through the creation of a seated audience section using a streamer or long stretch of fabric indicating the stage line. Participants then configured themselves in an opening circle for an embodied check-in. Each week, the play space was concretized in the same way. Ending the session also involved repeated practices, indicating re-entry from the dramatic into real time and space. These included necessary grounding, a reflection space, a return to the circle for a final check-out and a ritualized closure of the space that acknowledged group connection. Grounding rituals offered a transitional space between inner and outer realms of experience (Smail, 2013). These involved directed engagement with one's own physical body and/or material objects in the room. These grounding rituals were constructed as a game, i.e. *'touch this to that ...'* or movement practice, *'stamp your feet, shake your arms'*, which retained group playfulness whilst increasing participant's awareness of their physical body in relationship to surroundings.

Holding a reflection space for participants to integrate their experiences, invited shared insight about what could be useful in real life. This reflection space was described by adolescent participants as important:

*'We don't often get asked what we think'*

*'Or treated like teenagers'*

*'Dramatherapy is a more mature group. We get to say what we really think and feel ... Everyone gets to have their turn, to have their say and everyone has to listen'.*

(Musicka-Williams, 2020a)

Inclusion of a final check-out through gesture ensured everyone could make a contribution and have their response witnessed in the reflection space.

Following closing procedures, the space returned to classroom normalcy. Ritualized routines enabled participants to take lead and ownership over entrances and exits into the dramatic space. They symbolized a bridging space between real life and the world of one's creation, making sought-after adolescent rites of passage accessible to participants who felt they were denied such opportunities to construct their own realities in ways that their adolescent peers without disabilities were not.

### Relational Space

In concluding a discussion of essential conceptualizations of space and the related factors which serve to define the dramatherapy space in special education, the importance of fostering a healthy relational space is discussed. The dramatic arts offer unique spaces of social inclusion and belonging for people living with disabilities (Bailey, 2010, 2018; Ineland and Sauer, 2016; Lister *et al.*, 2009). Drama and creative processes allow for unique self-expression and ways of inter-relating. In dramatherapy, we offer practical pathways for shared creativity which acknowledge the intersubjective nature of human experience (Pitruzzella, 2017).

This final section explores the ways in which dramatherapy invites young people in special education to co-create a relational space through dramatic interaction. Specific consideration is given to how we dramatically explore and sustain a relational space that honours interdependency, an experience which often defines the relational lives of people living with disabilities (Reindal, 1999).

### Self and Other in Space

Recognition of one's own physical self in space is fundamental to dramatic play (Dokter, 2016; Jennings, 2011). An embodied, dramatic experience of the self includes recognition of body boundaries and awareness of one's physical self in relationship to surrounding people and environments (Booker, 2011). Recognition of one's self as actively and playfully engaged with another human in space constitutes an important developmental awareness (Jennings, 2011). Furthermore, such encounters reflect how the reality of human existence is constructed from a series of dramatic and intersubjective experiences that we actively co-create alongside others (Pitruzzella, 2017). Playful encounters invite engagement with all domains of human experience, our senses, emotional responses, capacity for dialogue and cognitive reflection, in responsiveness to shared realities.

Much of dramatherapy practice in special education meets students at stages of development, where awareness of self is developing. Therefore, recognition of self and others in shared spaces and interactions represents a fundamental therapeutic goal. This goal is addressed through offering dramatherapy as a means of multimodal engagement with self and others. Multimodality offers a developmentally accessible process and an enticing invitation to play (Porter, 2017).

## Play Space of the Body

The following vignette describes work with a young man whose developing awareness of body boundaries in relationship to space was explored as a basis from which to establish relational awareness. Max was presented as a potential participant for a short-term project focused on developing relational skills. An adolescent, Max was non-verbal and diagnosed with severe intellectual disability and autism. Beginning to explore an extended sense of his own physical capacities, Max demonstrated limited tolerance for engaging with others, except at times where he required personal care assistance. Engaging Max in dramatherapy involved a stripping down of the dramatic process to intensive interaction like play. In constructing a therapeutic approach to suit Max's needs, I drew upon my training in the Sesame approach to drama and movement therapy, which emphasizes indirect, symbolic and often non-verbal, movement-based practice which incorporates therapeutic use of touch (Lindvisk, 1997; Pearson, 1996; Porter, 2014). In consultation with the teaching staff, the goals were to increase Max's sense of bodily awareness and responsiveness to others.

In setting up a dramatherapy space, it was apparent I would need to work with Max wherever I found him. This was sometimes in the classroom, either empty or with others, and sometimes in the surrounding gardens where he immersed himself in a sensory experience. Initially, I attempted to define the dramatherapy space with a few simple props. These became projectiles. Only after many sessions spent establishing rapport did Max begin to use them in cause and effect co-operative play.

I came to realize that it was our bodies in space, their proximity to one another, the use of touch and the bearing of physical weight that would create a potential space where Max could playfully re-experience himself in relationship to another (Winnicott, 1971). I used my voice to create and hold space to establish a sense of interpersonal connection in a way that was developmentally appropriate, incorporating rhyme and rhythm as cues for self-recognition and relational engagement (Jennings, 2011). I sang instructions to Max about what I was doing and about the different parts of his physical self that were engaged in play. I demonstrated our connectedness and separateness through weight bearing and gestural play (Loutsis, 2017) in both co-active and turn-taking tasks. Our physical bodies were the primary definers of the dramatic space and the central focus of practice. As Max's awareness of his body grew, he began to reach out, to tolerate and begin to play with my presence. Entrance into dramatic play was scaffolded over time, emphasizing a mutual interdependence and co-active creativity which authentically reflected the lived experience of Max as a young person living with complex disability (Booker, 2011).

## Conclusion

Within this chapter, an argument has been presented for why 'space' and participant's multifaceted relationship to it are pivotal in enabling the unique experience that dramatherapy offers to young people in special education.

I have defined what I have found in practice to be four essential conceptualizations of space which influence meaningful engagement with dramatherapy for participants with intellectual/developmental disabilities. These include broad consideration of physical, psychological, imaginal and relational space factors. As a dramatherapist in special education, my personal and professional relationship to space, the way I think about and relate to it, and its inhabitants, has been influenced by the diversity experienced in this setting. When I reflect on my experiences alongside participants of dramatherapy in special education, I realize how personal and how fundamentally creative our interactions with space are. In dramatherapy, I witness the unique and surprising ways in which young people with intellectual/ developmental disabilities engage with the therapeutic space, and I know then that my own definition and experiences of space will never adequately explain the experiences of the young people in this setting. I must choose instead to continually re-enter the play space, to re-negotiate it and to re-experience the dramatherapy space according to what each young person brings into and through it.

## References

Allan, J. (2014) 'Inclusive education and the arts', *Cambridge Journal of Education*, 44(4), pp. 511–523.

Anaby, D., Hand, C., *et al.* (2013) *Disability and Rehabilitation*, 35(19), pp. 1589–1598.

Bailey, S. (2010) *Barrier-Free Theatre*. USA: Idyll Arbor.

Bailey, S., Burr, B., *et al.* (2018) 'Making an Inclusive Community Through Inclusive, Barieer Free Theatre', *North American Drama Therapy Association Conference, October 2018*. Kansas City: Kansas State University, pp. 1–19.

Booker, M. (2011) *Developmental Drama*. London: Jessica Kingsley Publishers.

Cassidy, S., Gurnely, A., *et al.* (2017) 'Safety, play, enablement, and active involvement: Themes from a grounded theory study of practitioner and client experiences of change processes in dramatherapy', *The Arts in Psychotherapy*, 55, pp. 174–185.

Cassidy, S., Turnbull, S., *et al.* (2014) 'Exploring core processes facilitating therapeutic change in dramatherapy: A grounded theory analysis of published case studies', *The Arts in Psychotherapy*, 41(4), pp. 353–365.

Chesner, A. (1995) *Dramatherapy for People with Learning Disabilities: A World of Difference*. London & Philadelphia: Jessica Kingsley Publishers.

Crimmens, P. (2006) *Drama Therapy and Storymaking in Special Education*. London & Philadelphia: Jessica Kingsley Publishers.

Curtis, S. (2016) *Space, Place and Mental Health*. London: Routledge.

Dokter, D. (2016) 'Embodiment in Dramatherapy', in Jennings, S. and Holmwood, C. (eds.) *Routledge International Handbook of Dramatherapy*. London & New York: Routledge, pp. 115–124.

Dunne, P. (2009) 'Narradrama: A Narrative Approach to Drama Therapy', in Johnson, D.R. and Emunah, R. (eds.) *Current Approaches in Drama Therapy*. Illinois: Charles C. Thomas Publishers, pp. 172–204.

Gaspar, T., Bilimoria, H., *et al.* (2016) 'Children with special education needs and subjective well-being: Social and personal influence', *International Journal of Disability, Development and Education*, 63(5), pp. 500–513.

Goodley, D., Runswick-Cole, K. and Liddiard, K. (2016) 'The dishuman child', *Discourse: Studies in the Cultural Politics of Education*, 37(5), pp. 770–774.

Holmwood, C. (2014) *Drama Education and Dramatherapy: Exploring the Space between Disciplines.* London & New York: Routledge.

Ineland, J.I. and Sauer, L. (2016) 'Institutional environments and subcultural belonging: Theatre and intellectual disabilities', *Scandinavian Journal of Intellectual Disabilities*, 9(1), pp. 46–57.

Jennings, S. (2011) *Healthy Attachments and Neuro-Dramatic Play.* London & Philadelphia: Jessica Kingsley Publisher.

Jones, P. (2009) *Rethinking Childhood: Attitudes in Contemporary Society.* London & New York: Continuum.

Jones, P. (2016) 'How Do Dramatherapists Understand Client Change?', in Jennings, S. and Holmwood, C. (eds.) *Routledge International Handbook of Dramatherapy.* London & New York: Routledge, pp. 77–91.

Jones, P. and Elmer, S. (2019) 'Perspectives on Play: Learning for Life', in Brock, A., Jarvis, P. and Oulsoga, Y. (eds.) *Perspectives on Play: Learning for Life.* London & New York: Routledge, pp. 290–312.

Johnson, D.R. (2009) 'Developmental Transformations: Towards the Body as Presence', in Johnson, D.R. and Emunah, R. (eds.) *Current Approaches in Dramatherapy.* 2nd ed. Springfield: Charles C Thomas, pp. 89–116.

Landy, R.J. (1993) *Persona and Performance: The Meaning of Role in Drama, Therapy and Everyday Life.* London & Bristol: Jessica Kingsley Publishers.

Lindvisk, B. (1997) *Bring White Beads When You Call Upon the Healer.* New Orleans: Rivendell House.

Lister, S., Tanguay, D., Snow, S. and D'Amico, M. (2009) 'Development of a creative arts therapies center for people with developmental disabilities', *Art Therapy*, pp. 34–37.

Loutsis, A. (2017) 'Body, Movement and Trauma', in Hougham, R. and Jones, B. (eds.) *Dramatherapy: Reflections and Praxis.* London: Palgrave.

Mussa, A. (2016) '"I Am a Black Flower" the Use of Rituals in Dramatherapy Work with a Special Education Class in Arab-Israeli Society', in Jennings, S. and Holmwood, C. (eds.) *Routledge International Handbook of Dramatherapy: (208-2017).* London: Routledge.

Musicka-Williams, A. (2020a) *No innovation without imitation: Using group dramatherapy to explore relationships and interpersonal learning processes with adolescents in special education*, Minerva-access.unimelb.edu.au. http://hdl.net/11343/258585

Musicka-Williams, A. (2020b) '"We copy to join in, to not be lonely": Adolescents in special education reflect on using dramatic imitation in group dramatherapy to enhance relational connection and belonging', *Frontiers in Psychology*, 11, p. 588650.

Pearson, J. (1996) 'Discovering the Self', in Pearson, J. (ed.) *Discovering the Self Through Drama and Movement.* London & New York: Jessica Kingsley Publishers, pp. 7–16.

Pendzik, S. (2006) 'On dramatic reality and its therapeutic function in drama therapy', *Arts in Psychotherapy*, 33(4), pp. 271–280.

Pitruzzella, S. (2017) *Drama, Creativity and Intersubjectivity.* London & New York: Routledge.

Porter, R. (2014) 'Movement with touch and sound in the Sesame approach: Bringing bones to the flesh', *Dramatherapy*, 36(1), pp. 27–42.

Porter, R. (2017) 'Multimodality', in Hougham, R. and Jones, B. (eds.) *Dramatherapy: Reflections and Praxis*. London: Palgrave, pp. 169–188.

Reindal, S.M. (1999) 'Independence, dependence, interdependence: Some reflections on the subject and personal autonomy', *Disability & Society*, 14(3), pp. 353–367.

Roger, J. (2012) 'Learning Disabilities and Finding, Protecting and Keeping the Therapeutic Space', in Leigh, L., Gerch, I., Dix, A. and Haythorne, D. (eds.) *Dramatherapy with Children, Young People and Schools*. Hove, East Sussex: Routledge, pp. 129–135.

Sajnani, N. (2016) 'How acting as if can make a dramatic difference', *Drama Therapy Review*, 2(2), pp. 163–166.

Smail, M. (2013) 'Entering and Leaving the Place of Myth', in Pearson, J., Smail, M. and Watts, P. (eds.) *Dramatherapy with Myth and Fairytale: The Golden Stories of Sesame*. London: Jessica Kingsley Publishers, pp. 55–72.

Winnicott, D. (1971) *Playing and Reality*. London & New York: Routledge.

Part 3

# Ritual, Intersubjective and Spiritual Space

*Eliza Sweeney*

# 8 The Fullness of Emptiness

## The Significance of Space and the Usefulness of the Concepts of *Shunya* (The Void/Empty Space), *Akasha* or *Vyoman* (Open Vastness), *Kha* (The Enclosed Space) in Hinduism and Buddhism for Dramatherapy Practice

*Bruce Howard Bayley*

The material I have chosen for this chapter is located within the context of an approach that I have developed and designated as Tribhuvan Threefold Psycho-spiritual Dramatherapy (http://www.brucebayley.co.uk/trib-bhb.htm) that takes a psycho-spiritual and transpersonal perspective informed by a variety of spiritual traditions including Vedanta, Ayurveda, Buddhist and Taoist texts and art and Goethean psychology and concepts from Rudolf Steiner's Spiritual Science. Raising questions relating to some of the perspectives on Space within dramatherapy, my intention is to focus on notions of Space from within these traditions and their usefulness in dramatherapy practice. Commencing with a brief consideration of Space in theatre and therapy, I will present notions of inner, outer and liminal space. I will offer a chance to ponder on some of our existing perceptions of Space and Time and I shall look at aspects of *Śunya* (the void/space), *Akhaśa* or *Vyoman* (the open vastness) and *Kha* (the enclosed space), which is represented by the cave, as they are presented within Vedatta and Buddhism. I will be referring to illustrative examples from my dramatherapy practice that considers the processes of focusing inwards, emptying out and opening up by creating, emptying and re-creating afresh within the therapeutic space. The intrinsic relation in Buddhism between *Shunya* (empty space) and *Karuna* (compassion) signifies the essential inter-relatedness of things in the phenomenal world and leads me to further reflect on the value (fullness) of the empty space, seeking to articulate the relevance of these ideas and images for dramatherapy practice.

For the reader note that I will be using the capital letter S when I am referring to the concept of *Space* and the lower case 's' when referring to specific space/spaces as locations – *the dramatherapy space, the space between us, theatre space, etc.* I also use the upper-case letters 'G' and 'B' when I refer to proper nouns and concepts such as *Ground of Being*, *God* and *Being* and the lower-case letters 'g' and 'b' for common nouns and internal words such as

DOI: 10.4324/9781003252399-12

*god* or a human *being*. I will be using the form *sh* in place of the sign indicating the palatal hard letter *ś* in the spellings of *Akasha* and *Shunya*.

## The Question of Space in Dramatherapy Practice

If it is true that at the heart of dramatherapy practice, there is some change sought by client and therapist alike through dynamic, expressive and psychological interchanges which, when reflected on and acknowledged, will bring insight, healing or transformation, then within this notion I see questions relating to identity and also to the location:

- Who or what is to change?
- Where does the process take place?
- What relationship does the client/therapist have to the space? How does the client's/therapist's relationship with the space contribute to the process?
- May liminal spaces be considered to be useful or not in facilitating the therapy process?

The ethno-historian Greg Dening approaches the question of ideas, theatre and space by referring to them as *sets*. He writes in *Performances* (1996) that:

> 'Theory' and 'theatre' come to us out of the same Greek origin – *thea*, sight, viewing; *theoros*, spectator. Theory - a mind-set for viewing; theatre - a space-set for spectatoring; theatrical - a convention-set for *mimesis*.
> (Dening, 1996: 104)

If we are to devise a way of seeing this place of viewing, then the questions 'What do we mean by Space?' and 'What is this Space?' become fundamental. The space in which the event takes place is a prime signifier of the event. Its shape, size and structure affect the dynamic relationship between all the participants to the point where the question 'What space is it?' is certainly worth considering. The physical body, presence, mental and emotional states of being and actions of the performer/s would be fundamental aspects of this 'convention-set', just as any location at which the performance would be taking place – a theatre, a cabaret bar, a street corner or a park – would be a valid 'space-set'. These questions with regard to theatre can also be extended to pondering the issues of space in dramatherapy. The mindsets of participants (clients and therapists), their emotional states, their perspectives, their expectations and how they view the transformational processes of healing or ritual within the therapy and the space in which it takes place will have fundamental effects on themselves, their journeys and the outcomes of the therapy. As will the nature, shape, structure, quality and atmosphere of the space itself. How we view ideas about Space and location will derive largely from which of the prevalent world views we choose to adopt.

With the arrival of the novel coronavirus in 2019, the ensuing epidemic and the lengthy worldwide lockdowns that have followed, we have seen an increase in online therapy and supervision sessions. With it have come both benefits and challenges to notions relating to the nature of the therapy space. I am not seeking to discuss these here but I will be raising some questions about them at the end of this chapter. I am simply acknowledging that they have necessarily impacted and influenced traditional views that have been held regarding space in dramatherapy practice.

## Therapeutic Space and Sacred Space

In her consideration of sacred spaces, Susana Pendzik (1994) distinguishes sacred space from the non-sacred by virtue of its enclosed nature and boundary that acts as a 'consciously devised protective tool that temporarily eliminates anxieties and fears by preventing the shadow archetype from entering into the enclosed area' (1994: 29). She compares the therapeutic space to the sacred space:

> The parallels between sacred and therapeutic spaces are too many to be undermined or attributed to coincidence. Like the function of the circle, other aspects of the sacred space need to be investigated so that the archetype's hidden wisdom is re-discovered and its therapeutic potential effectively used.
>
> (Pendzik, 1994: 30)

In *Ritual and Theatre* (2014), Roger Grainger establishes how ritual marks the passage of time and that it does so by:

> using metaphors of geographical extension in which we clear a space within the flow of time in order to make contact with the source of being and become changed receiving the necessary ability to embark on a new and unknown phase of life.
>
> (Grainger, 2014: 78)

In considering significant sacred spaces such as shrines, Grainger points out that they need not be fixed in any specific location as we have the ability to create or re-create a focused awareness of a 'presence beyond the limitations of space and time' (Ibid: 80) wherever we wish to be. One level at which I see therapy operating is in providing some kind of healing process for disease in which the therapist facilitates the client to access the self-healing resources that lie within themselves from which the client (as well as therapist) may be disconnected – a spiritual resource, if I may use that word without seeming to exoticize or *magicalize* it. The language and terminology employed in Depth Psychology and the invitations to clients to visualize their inner landscapes, to process their wounded inner children or to employ a degree of aesthetic distancing that invokes established notions of inner (subjective) and outer (objective) spaces are pertinent here. Such notions of inner and outer space with liminal threshold spaces in between them are informed by particular perceptions and expectations of locality and consciousness. Other perceptions and expectations have been held over the centuries by the metaphysical and spiritual-scientific work of poets, thinkers, scientists and philosophers such as Blake, Swedenborg, Schiller, Goethe and Rudolf Steiner in the West as well as by traditional cosmological philosophies of Hinduism, Buddhism and Taoism, for instance.

Eben Alexander, the famous American neurosurgeon, following his near-death experience in 2008, writes in great detail in *Proof of Heaven* (2012) about his direct experience of different levels of consciousness under medically induced coma that led him to a total reappraisal of the world view held by him and of his life's work as a neuroscientist. My own experience of a threshold consciousness following life-or-death surgery in 2015, when the surgeons had informed me that I may only have had two days to live, led to a similar reappraisal of my own work in dramatherapy. I had also already been acquainted with the ground breaking explorative work of Isabel Clarke, consultant clinical psychologist in acute mental health in the Hampshire Partnership NHS Foundation Trust (Clarke, 2010), in the psychology of psychosis and spirituality, and was aware of the UK Spiritual Crisis Network begun by Catherine Lucas in 2004. Both of these were inspirational to me in the development of my series of workshops *Dramatherapy and the New Paradigm* in 2013 which then developed into my current work *Tribhuvan Threefold Psycho-spiritual Dramatherapy* (http://www.brucebayley.co.uk/tribhuvan_threefold_dramatherapy.pdf. Accessed June 2017).

Eben Alexander writes:

We have been seduced into thinking that the scientific world view is fast approaching a Theory of Everything (TOE), which would not seem to leave much room for our soul ... !

(Alexander, 2012: 153)

At the heart of the enigma of quantum mechanics lies the falsehood of our notion of locality in space and time ... The entire length and height of the physical universe is as nothing to the spiritual realm from which it has arisen – the realm of consciousness (which some might refer to as 'the life force').

(Ibid: 155–156)

Alexander's reference to the 'spiritual realm' and the 'life force' from which the physical universe 'has arisen' leads me to consider the importance of considering other perceptions/notions of space and locality and the nature of states of consciousness (which some may refer to us *stages* or *realms*) in dramatherapy practice.

## Space and Locality in Hindu and Buddhist Traditions: *Akasha/Vyoman*; *Shunya* and *Kha*

Before going on to look at the implications of these views of Space for Dramatherapy and some of the ways which illustrate their uses in practice, I will offer a necessary but brief look at *Akasha* (the open vastness or ether), *Shunya* (the empty or void Space) and *Kha* (the enclosed space or cavity) within Vedanta and Buddhism.

### Akasha *and* Vyoman – *The Upper Sky, The Ether, The Open Vastness*

The *Upanishads* are traditional Sanskrit texts that form the foundations of Vedanta. They are of uncertain authorship, composed between 2 and 3 millennia ago, and present philosophical questions in an archaic, mystical and ritual context. In *From the Upanishads* (1996), Dr Ananda Wood follows the Advaita Vedanta tradition as interpreted by Sri Atmananda Krishna Menon. Wood's translation of the key idea in the Chandogya Upanishad is as follows: 'what is this change and movement that appears to form our world? ... All moving things and changing forms arise, take shape, continue on and come to end in space alone' (Wood, 1996: 101).

Here Wood is using the word 'space' as a translation of the word *Akasha* which also means sky or ether and which Robert Svoboda, the Ayurvedic practitioner, teacher and writer, refers to as being one of the 'Five Great Elements' in the system of Ayurveda (Svoboda, 1993: 45), the other four being earth, air, fire and water. The concept of Space here is an all-embracing one containing everything. Wood refers to this as not 'a narrow sense as the distance that separates objects' but as a universal pervasiveness, as 'continuing space and time' (Wood, 1996: 101). Space (*Akasha*) is the source of everything, contains everything and is also the end of everything. This concept of *Akasha* seems to correspond to that presented in the New Testament of the Bible in the words of St Paul before the Areopagus, where God is described as a Being in whom 'we live, move and have our being' (Acts 17:28, KJV), and who is referred to within Christian Existentialism as the (Divine) 'Ground of Being'. Paul Tillich, the German-American Christian existential philosopher, and Lutheran Protestant theologian present this view of God as 'Being' itself, the 'Ground of Being' and the 'power of Being' where God is seen as being beyond essence and existence (Tillich, 1951: 235–236). Wood goes on to suggest that there is a sense here that is akin to Einstein's theory of relativity with the conception of the physical world as a space–time continuum in which everything – space, matter, time and energy - is essentially inter-related and must be taken together. This is a world where there is no separation between the object and the observer or the experiment from the experimenter. Eben Alexander points to this being a major factor in understanding the spiritual realm and the relationship between consciousness and physical reality that is at the heart of quantum mechanics. He goes on to suggest that this is a far more mysterious revelation than physicists and neuroscientists have shown themselves capable of dealing with, and their failure to do so has left the intimate relationship between consciousness and quantum mechanics obscured.

(Alexander, 2012: 154)

*Akasha* may also be understood as being the upper sky, the big sky over mountain peaks or the vast openness over wide, flat plains – the nature of which gives rise to yearnings for freedom and almost ancient callings of worlds beyond us. This apparent empty vastness is not vacant but full of everything. In *From the Upanishads* (1996), Wood writes:

'space' is not here conceived in a narrow sense as the distance that *separates* particular objects. Instead, it is conceived in a more universal sense as *continuing* space and time which together contain the entire universe, and which thus *connect* different objects.

(Wood, 1996: 101)

*Vyoman* is a Sanskrit word having similar meanings to *Akasha*, varying from heaven, sky, atmosphere, ether and water to signify more specific locations such as a temple sacred to the Sun and the home of Lord Vishnu. In modern usage, the word *vyomanaut* is used for an Indian astronaut or someone working on India's space programme. Unlike *Akasha*, however, *Vyoman* also has a personified form of Lord Shiva. In Tagare's translation of *The Skanda Purana* (one of the religious texts composed in Sanskrit from the 2nd CE), we read:

Śiva is the Lord without beginning and end.

He is the greatest *Vyoman*.

There is none greater than he.

(Tagare, 1950, *7.1.10.17*).

### Shunya – *The Empty Space, The Void Space*

In Sanskrit, the word *shunya* means zero – nothing. It is the root in the word *shunyata* – meaning emptiness or nothingness – and is itself derived from the root word *svi* (hollow). *Shunya* and *Shunyata* both appear within the texts of Buddhism as well as those of different Hindu denominations. There are, however, variations as to emphasis in meaning and implication. In Buddhist philosophy, *Shunya*, the void space, is a constituent of the state known as Shunyata and is usually translated as emptiness or hollowness. It is not to be seen as a negation that would give it a nihilistic quality which would be to misunderstand it.

In some texts of Shaivite Hinduism (devotion to the Lord Shiva), *Shunya* as voidness is mentioned as a feature of ultimate reality. In Jaideva Singh's

*Vijnanabhairava* or Divine Consciousness (1979), *Lord Shiva* (also known by other names such as *Bhairava* and *Rudra*) is called the 'Absolute Void', beyond all categories:

'From the point of view of the human mind, He is most void. From the point of view of Reality, He is most full, for He is the source of all manifestation'.

(Singh, 1979: 29)

In the texts of Vaishnavism (devotion to *Lord Vishnu*), *Shunya* is presented as a personified Void known as *Shunya Purusha*, bringing it closer to the concept of *Brahman* than to the view held of *Shunyata* in Buddhism (Dalal, 2010: 388–389), *Brahman* being the ultimate reality, the unity that binds all Diversity. In this respect, it seems similar to the concept of *Akasha*.

There are parallel notions to *Shunya* in Taoism known as *Wu* (nothingness) or *Hsu* (vacant). Apart from being central and fundamental concepts in the philosophies of Buddhism and Taoism, *Shunya* and *Wu* (or *Hsu*) are also significant for the aesthetics of both traditions, for we need to consider the extent to which the arts reflect the spirit and the consciousness of religions.

### Kha – *The Enclosed Space, The Cavity, The Cave, The Grotto*

This is the enclosed space – where the empty space invites us to move inwards and look into or enter a cavity, a cave or a grotto. Here again, this is not necessarily vacant or negative but a secreted internal space – an intimate space associated with the heart. Enclosed spaces have traditionally been seen as sacred spaces (the Buddhist cave temples at Ellora, Ajanta and the Karla Caves in Maharashtra, India), but also as mysterious, secret, hidden storage spaces for contraband goods (smugglers' caves in Cornwall), as reclusive spaces for hermits, anchorite monks and nuns (such as Mother Julian the fourteenth-century anchorite's small walled up room attached to a church in Norwich), or as sites for divine encounters or apparitions (the grotto at Lourdes).

Many of these enclosed spaces are to be found in natural land formations. However, many of them are created by digging or hollowing out rocky terrain, digging into the land or being erected by building materials to form cells. Art and Aesthetics researcher Sung-Min Kim describes this emptying process in regard to the art of cave temples in *Śunya: Immanent and Transcendent: Investigating Meanings of Void* (2007):

The creation of a cave temple starts from the act of digging gross rock materials. The pure void is unveiled and revealed as the rock materials are removed. The further creative chiselling brings forth embellishing forms along with the cavity. In other words, the essential process of excavation is to recover a form latent in gross materials by means of 'emptying'.

(Kim, 2007: 33)

There is some sense here of poeisis, the kind of making/creating that Martin Heidegger in *The Origin of the Work of Art* (1956) refers to as a 'bringing-forth' (*Basic Writings*, 2008: 118) in its widest sense – bringing something from a hidden state into the full light of a created work, a process of 'unveiling', a threshold occasion when something moves away from being one thing to become another or where something is removed. In *Poiesis and Art-Making: A Way of Letting-Be* (2003), Derek Whitehead writes:

> The Greeks drew a distinction between poiesis and praxis. Praxis in the Greek sense had to do with the immediate sense of 'an act', of a will that accomplishes or completes itself in action. Poiesis was conceived as bringing something from concealment into the full light and radiation of a created work. Poiesis is not to be grasped in its features as a practical or voluntary activity, but rather in its being an 'unveiling', a-letheia.
>
> (Whitehead, 2003)

A major personal interest for me in my dramatherapy practice lies in facilitating these two processes of unveiling/revealing and filling/emptying. I have used specific enactment interventions based on the processes of filling and emptying space at various points during dramatherapy sessions depending on the presenting issues and emerging needs of clients which I will illustrate here.

*Illustrations from Dramatherapy Practice*

---

**Vignette 1**

**Example within group sessions – filling and emptying the external space (*Kha* and *Shunya*)**

The group was made up of eight university students halfway through a ten-month Group Dramatherapy journey. For a number of weeks, several members of the group had been bringing their anger and frustrations to the sessions. The university year was nearing its closure and some students were beginning to feel that they were not being given enough support in assisting them to manage what they had begun to identify as 'overload'. One of the members was going through problems in her personal life and she had asked for more time to hand in an assignment which had not been granted. Her tempestuous feelings were in control of her and she was acting out in a belligerent manner using vivid lavatorial language. Other members of the group were trying to manage her without having an effect. The process of expressing anger and frustration was mounting in belligerent shouting and gestures until a member who had been passive up till this point was suddenly aroused out of his silence. He stood up and shouted, 'This is all a pile of crap!' He looked at me as if he wanted me to intervene. I suggested that this might be a valuable point in the group's journey and invited them to trash the room by taking all the objects they could find in the room – paper, pencils, paints and furniture – and making a pile in the middle of the room. They tore the paper. They upturned the chairs, tables, cushions, curtains, musical instruments, drapes and noticeboards. They were beginning to look like a small but rebellious crowd. They strewed all the pens, pencils and pastels over the floor and didn't stop until there was a large mound comprising a variety of objects and materials in the middle of the otherwise empty space. Then they laughed and laughed. I asked them to form a circle around the dump and simply look at their creation in silence. Gradually, as if waking up from a frenzy, the group took on a different form and atmosphere. They became very quiet and some of them seemed to appear to be embarrassed as they took their places on the ground around the pile in the middle of the circular space in the room.

The dramatherapy space had almost taken on the qualities of a sacred space and reflected a temple-like quality with the participants sitting around the mound resembling a group of attendants at a ritual ceremony. The room itself had the elements of *Kha,* being an enclosed space within which the group had created a round shape of a mound out of the materials and objects that they had used to express their initial rage. The space surrounding the mound – between it and the high ceiling of the room – formed a void shape, reminiscent of *Shunya.* The space in the room, the curved shape of the mound within the Void and the members sitting in a ritual circle around the mound had taken on the ritual quality reminiscent of the interior meditation hall of a Buddhist cave temple such as at Karla in Maharashtra, India (see Figure 8.1.)

Within the silence, the group members experienced different feelings and reactions and went through different actions. After substantial reflection, they became very serious and expressed many emotions – relief, shame, embarrassment as well as joy. After a while, the initial rage began to turn into an urge to put everything back. I suggested that they do so in as ritualistic a manner as they could while reflecting on each article that they were moving. When they had done this, I invited them again to sit in silence and look at the empty space in front of us. They were very quiet and two of the members became tearful. They closed the session saying that they felt very moved.

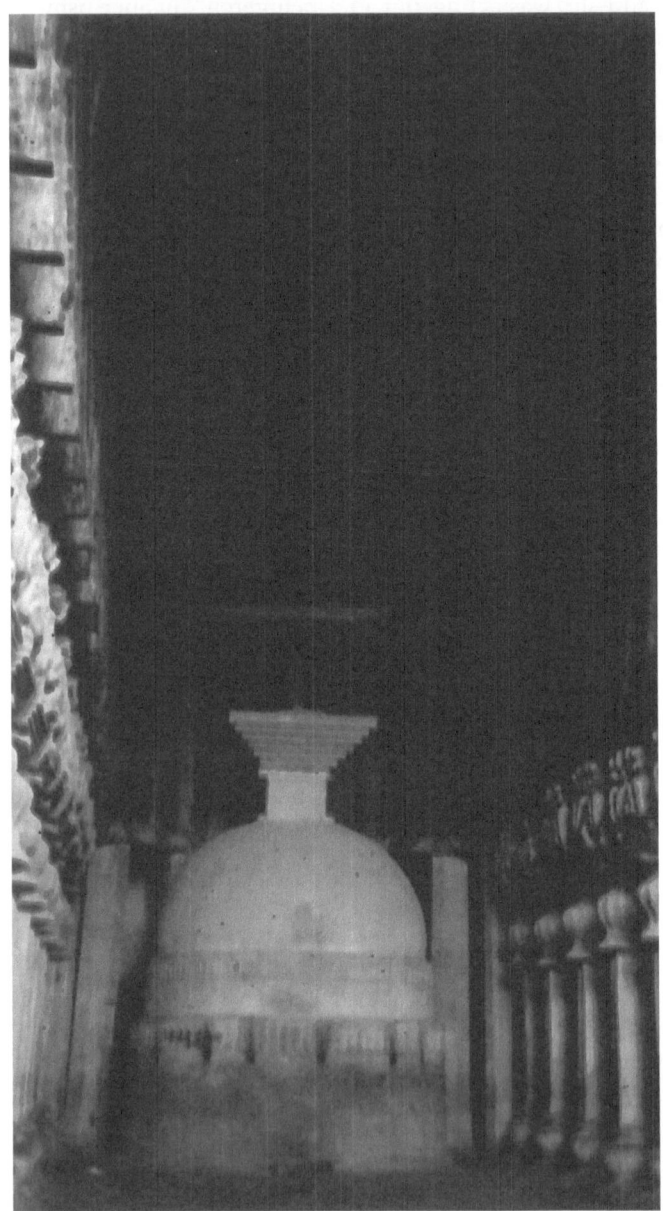

*Figure 8.1* Meditation hall, Karla temple cave, Maharashtra, India (Photograph by Bruce Howard Bayley).

After this session, the group turned a corner. The trashing process had filled the room with all their projected frustrations and rage in a very real way – not simply symbolic, and the fully trashed space reflected the internal chaos of their group psyche back to them. The trashing process allowed them to express their internal rage which ended in relief and joy, but it was the emptying of the space and the subsequent contemplation of the emptiness that had resulted in something shifting for them, individually as well as collectively. Their response to what they had perceived as badness had left them with a resultant sense of felt badness – but only temporarily. In their reflection of the emptiness, the badness had metamorphosed into a sense of newness wherein something else could then be contemplated. The members were able then to move on. While the experience was focused on the external space (the room and its objects), the process undertaken was also an internal one of inner psychic decluttering as well. It was as if the silent contemplation of the empty *Shunya* (void) had provided them with the opportunity to open a space within themselves and begin to enter inner spaces with qualities that were different from the feelings that they had been full of previously – resentment, anger and rage had begun to give way to tender feelings that were now accessing them to reconsider and feel more able to tolerate the situations which had made them feel powerless previously – as if they had taken a journey from states of anger to states of acceptance via the changes within the emptiness of the *Shunya* space.

**Vignette 2**

**Example from individual sessions – clearing the internal space (*Kha*)**

Client Y was a woman in her thirties who had had a significant period in her teenage years of early sexual experiences with a family friend who was also one of her father's work colleagues. She had been struggling with the memory of the abuse because she was conflicted as to whether or not she had been complicit in agreeing to the sexual encounters whereby she had derived a degree of pleasure. This inner conflict had left her with a restlessness that she felt in her adult relationships with intimate partners, which she described as a 'push me-pull you' dynamic. The memories of the sexual abuse had led her to feel increasingly conflicted between rage and guilt. She said that she had felt 'full of rubbish' and 'unclean, filthy' – as if she wanted to purge.

She performed a series of enactments over a number of weeks in which she developed a character who strode about the space in a series of dance movements which evoked the feeling of a woman seeking revenge, appearing to brandish weapons in the air and making seductive-looking strides. The vengeful character developed into one that she called the 'Water Spout' in which she puffed her body out, blowing her lips and mouth and contorting her limbs. So began the process of emptying out the enclosed internal chambers (*Kha*) of her lungs, throat, heart and abdomen. She took on the characteristics of an enraged balloon and then she began belching, vomiting motions as she crossed the external space of the room in large strides. This work also involved working with prana (breath) and the chakras (energy centres) which I refer to in my chapter *'Embodying Ramayana: the drama within'* in the *International Handbook of Dramatherapy* (eds: Jennings and Holmwood, 2017: 26–35). Each enactment lasted between 10 and 15 minutes until she had reached a point when she felt she had purged enough. At the end of each enactment, she expressed self-comforting sounds, smiling, breathing deeply and freely and saying that she had started to feel cleansed week after week. This formed a major intervention in the therapy process.

In Mahayana Buddhism, compassion is known as *Karuna* and connects with *Shunya* insofar as the quality of openness or of the emptiness of *Shunya* translates into acceptance. The act of digging out and emptying the earth or land in order to form the empty cave is itself a process whereby a new space is created, a virgin place, in which we can begin to consider new choices in order to begin to heal. Viewing *Shunya* in this way, Sung-Min Kim says, 'will help us to be free from the preconception that sees *Shunya* as a negative vacuum' (Kim, 2007: 36). It was the beginning of a process by which Y could begin to come to different ways of viewing and evaluating the past events. In a very different way from the group enactment of the trashing process, Y had been able to achieve a sense of feeling clean only after she had symbolically emptied the internal cavity (*Kha* space) formed by her stomach, chest, heart and throat areas. She said that this emptying process had enabled her to begin to renew her efforts at getting on with her life in a less traumatically triggered manner.

Working with *Akasha* and *Shunya* can enhance the ways by which we can access areas of feeling located around the Heart Centre. Yoga and meditation writer and teacher Michael A. Singer calls this working with one's 'inner energy' that can enable us to be able to acknowledge and express feelings such as love or compassion from which we may have previously been 'blocked'. In this way, he suggests, we are able to realize what he calls 'the untethered soul' and so begin to effect a change from a tight, closed-in attitude to one by which stress may be transformed into serenity and resentment into acceptance (Michael A. Singer, 2007: 41–47).

### Reflections

In *The Redemptive Centre of the Loving Heart* (2019), I wrote:

There tends to be a general suspicion of and resistance to accept that which is 'hidden' due to lack of so-called measurable validating evidence - therefore some reluctance to validate the 'unveiling' process in creative arts therapy. There is, too, the concentration on cognitive awareness and the need for cognitive acknowledgment by the patient/client of predicted 'outcomes' when we are more often than not involved in unconscious processes with clients.

(Bayley, 2019: 72)

In this chapter, I have attempted to articulate an approach in dramatherapy practice that seeks to give access to greater potentials for self-healing, self-knowledge and consciousness where good may come from the transformative process that is informed by reflecting on, embodying and experiencing inwardly and outwardly the nature and qualities of the Space itself – *Shunya* (the void/empty space), *Kha* (the enclosed cavity space) within *Akasha* (the all-containing and transpersonal space).

Writing this in the context of the COVID pandemic era, the question of online space arises. As far as online and remote dramatherapy goes, we may ask whether or not we find the challenges to be welcome. Certain fundamental questions have arisen with regard to new expectations of boundaries, notions of embodiment, relationship, visibility and space. If therapeutic space is a space of safety, then what happens to the notion of a safe, shared, confidential space when clients and therapists participate in virtual interchanges between representations of themselves and where the functions of the processes of the therapy are often largely determined not by the participants but by the technology? Is the virtual nature of the therapy space an enhancement of the therapy process or a denial of the significance of Space?

When we consider these notions of Space within dramatherapy, we may ask ourselves whether or not we may be able to access a greater variety of creative opportunities through which to address newer depths of awareness, insight and transformation by reviewing the established expectations, boundaries and traditions of our working culture as artists, therapists and health professionals.

## References

Alexander, E. (2012) *Proof of Heaven*. New York: Simon & Schuster.

Bayley, B.H. (2017) 'Embodying Ramayana: The Drama Within', in Jennings and Holmwood (eds.) *The Routledge International Handbook of Dramatherapy* (2017: 26–35).

Bayley, B.H. (2019) 'The Redemptive Centre of the Loving Heart', in *Love is in the Earth*. London: Almyrah Press.

Clarke, I. (2010) 'Psychosis and Spirituality Revisited: The Frontier is Opening Up!', in Clarke, I. (ed.) *Psychosis and Spirituality: Consolidating the New Paradigm*. Wiley-Blackwell.

Dalal, R. (2010) *Hinduism: An Alphabetical Guide*. Penguin.

Dening, G. (1996) *Performances*. University of Chicago Press.

Grainger, R. (2014) *Ritual and Theatre*. London: Austin Macauley Publishers Ltd.

Heidegger, M. (1956) *The Origin of the Work of Art*, in 'Poetry, Language, Thought', trans. Albert Hofstadter (London and Toronto: Harper and Row, Perennial Library, 1971: 17-39)) in *Basic Writings*. Part 4. Routledge (2008).

Kim, S. (2007) '*Śunya:* Immanent and Transcendent: Investigating Meanings of Void Through Art's Space', in Ray, H.P. (ed.) *Sacred Landscapes in Asia: Shared Traditions, Multiple Histories.* Manohar.

Pendzik, S. (1994) 'The theatre stage & the sacred space: A comparison', *The Arts in Psychotherapy,* 21(1), pp. 25–35.

Singer, M. (2007) *The Untethered Soul.* Oakland: New Harbinger and Noetic Books.

Singh, J. (1979) *Vijnanabhairava, Or Divine Consciousness: A Treasury of 112 Types of Yoga, Motilal Banarsidass*

Svoboda, R.E. (1993) *Ayurveda: Life, Health and Longevity.* Penguin.

Tagare, G.V. (1950) *The Skanda Purana.* Wisdom Library. https://www.wisdomlib.org/hinduism/book/the-skanda-purana/d/doc626797.html (accessed 13.6.2021)

Tillich, P. (1951) *Systematic Theology,* Vol. 1. University of Chicago Press.

Whitehead, D.H. (2003) *Poiesis and Art-Making: A Way of Letting-Be,* in 'Contemporary Aesthetics' vol 1 http://hdl.handle.net/2027/spo.7523862.0001.005 (accessed 13/06/2021)

Wood, A. (1996) *From the Upanishads.* Zen Publications (2007).

# 9 'Clear the Space. Claim the Space. Sanctify the Space'

## Intersubjectivity and Spirituality in Dramatherapy According to Roger Grainger

*Salvo Pitruzzella*

Revd. Roger Grainger (1934–2015) is one of the major theorists in the field of dramatherapy. His several books and articles are a quest for drama's profoundest principles, analyzing in detail the mysterious mechanisms presiding over theatre, ritual and children's dramatic play and showing how they connect with human nature. According to Grainger, the structure of drama has a healing potential in itself, being fundamentally modelled on ritual, and he emphasized that in order to understand these processes, the notion of space plays a central role. From a dramatic point of view, space is neither an inert entity, or an empty container for physical bodies to act. Rather, it is a vibrant and meaningful co-constructed microcosmos, created by human relationships and serving them, and endowed with a spiritual, ego-transcending value. The creation of such a space parallels in many ways the bond-making process in human beings: Grainger stressed the concept of *Betweenness,* the space that divides and connects in which I can *be with* the other while not *becoming* the other.

I maintain that Grainger's notion of space, which is theatrically and philosophically founded, can be a precious guide both to understand the healing power of dramatherapy and to refine its practical tools. Having had the privilege of meeting him in person, in this essay I will attempt a dialogue with this great soul, using as a guide a motto he often uttered in his workshops: 'Clear the space. Claim the space. Sanctify the space'.

### Does the Universe Have a Centre?

I would like to start my reflections with two stories, apparently very different from each other, yet each dealing, in its own way, with the notion of space. The first is a very short sketch, just a tiny slice of the bourgeoning basket of stories contained in Jaime De Angulo's celebrated *Indian Tales.* Here it is.

*Tras … tras … tras …* The road is long and the travelling hard. Father Bear's journey to the village of the Cranes has barely begun, but his family is already tired. His son, Fox Boy, has got the HA HAs since this morning, and

DOI: 10.4324/9781003252399-13

Antelope his wife has been carrying the little Quail all day long, while he was clearing the track. As the amethyst evening starts turning into a dark blue night, Bear spots a neat clearing in the woods and stops the family to camp for the night. He picks up the stones from the corner where they were planning to lay down and moves them to the middle of the clearing to set a campfire, while his wife arranges the sleeping places and the children play around, picking fruits and berries from the wood. When a good arrangement is done, they sit by the fire, cook their food and enjoy their supper, chatting and joking all the time. Then Father Bear puts out the fire, but before they all go to sleep, he looks around and starts saying:

> 'Good night, Mountains, you must protect us tonight. We are strangers but we are good people. We don't mean harm to anybody. Good night, Mister Pine Tree. We are camping under you. You must protect us tonight. Good night, Mister Owl. I guess this is your home where we are camped. We are good people, we are not looking for trouble, we are just traveling. Good night, Chief Rattlesnake. Good night, everyone. Good night, Grass People, we have spread our bed right on top of you. Good night, Ground, we are lying right on your face. You must take care of us, we want to live a long time'.

(De Angulo, 1953: 21)

While they are having their long-deserved sleep, I will tell you the second story, trying to keep my voice low not to disturb them. It is a fairly longer one, concerning the first explorations of the possibility of using drama as a therapy made by my friend and mentor Roger Grainger, which Roger himself told me quite a few years ago, when he came to Italy to lead a workshop for my dramatherapy students at the Arts Therapies Centre in Lecco.

Although it was only late November, the snow was storming over the city. In the evening after the workshop, we had supper together in the restaurant of the tiny hotel on the lakeside where we were lodging. The hotel was entitled, like many places in Lecco, to one of the many characters of Italy's national novel, Alessandro Manzoni's *I promessi sposi* (*The Bethrothed*), which is set in that otherwise quite nondescript industrial town of the North. Curiously enough, the character in question is one of the less amiable in the novel: Don Abbondio, the cowardly priest who surrenders the threats of the villain's henchmen, choosing the easier and less dangerous way, thus revealing the hypocrisy of the clergy. In the novel, he is contrasted by the towering figure of Fra' Cristoforo, the wandering monk, who had been a great sinner and then repented and risked his life to serve the humble and the oppressed.

If a more personal digression is permitted, I would like to add that I got rid of religion because of the former kind of priests. I was born in the mid-fifties in the opposite corner of Italy, the far south Sicily. Those were the times when the mafia was starting to take over and put their hands on the cities, with the complicity of the catholic politicians and the complacency of the local catholic hierarchies. 'E mafia e parrini si dettiru la manu' (Mafia and priests have shaken their hands) are the words of a folk song of those days. So, in my youth, I grew disgusted by the 'double moral' of the clergy, who preached love but did not refuse the sacraments to merciless bosses and vicious killers, and I abandoned my juvenile faith. Some ten years later, after the war-like attacks that had killed the two judges who had dared to defy the mafia, a great revolt against this apparently invincible power shook the island and also involved the Church, with many priests exposing themselves at the forefront and some even brutally killed. However, even though I understood that something had changed, it was too late for me to get acquainted again with my former religion, as in time I had moved my quest for spirituality to other territories. Therefore, it was quite unusual that the scholar I recognized as the most influential in developing my way of understanding dramatherapy – this plump, kind, smiling gentleman sitting in front of me – was actually a priest. While waiting for our soup to be served, I asked him how did he run into dramatherapy, and this is what he told me.

### A Room for Beauty

As a freshly ordained priest of the Church of England, Roger was assigned as a chaplain at Wakefield Psychiatric Hospital, a very old-fashioned place.

> For generations, the existence of such hospitals symbolised the imminence of chaos, not merely as an idea but an actual presence. The hospital demonstrated that chaos could be controlled by being contained.
>
> (Grainger, 2010: 17)

His role as a chaplain was quite a peculiar one: on the one hand, he was part of the institution and considered by the inmates as a member of the staff, albeit not with the same authority. On the other hand, he did not respond directly to the hospital's hierarchy, but to a different power, as he was funded directly from the Church. This special status allowed that people came to him asking for advice and support, but in a way totally out of the medical domain.

> I do not know myself whether mental sickness is a literal, medical sickness or a moral decision, something in which the word 'sickness' can only be used metaphorically (...). I only know that patients consult me because, as a priest, I am associated with the idea of the forgiveness of sins as a practical possibility.
>
> (Grainger, 1979: 59)

Forgiving entails recognizing the bright spark that lies deep into each person, unscathed by heavy layers of pain and despair that might cover it. You may call it the immortal soul, or the Buddha's nature, or Socrates' *Daimon*, or not call it at all. 'Mutual forgiveness of each vice/such are the Gates of

Paradise', William Blake had written. Different from judgement, forgiveness combats evil by doing good. And for these people, it could be a lucky chance to be considered human subjects rather than just be identified with their sickness.

> The expertise of the hospital, the array of therapeutic resources, not to mention the uncanny psychic omniscience of the psychiatrist himself (a man who knows what I'm thinking and why I'm thinking it, asking me questions to which he already knows the answers) tend to alert the patient's defences. (…) The chaplain, however, is not concerned to *get through to* the man or woman who comes to see him, but only to *be with* them.
>
> (Grainger, 1979: 39)

Right in the middle of the old building, the young new chaplain found the space that had been assigned to him by the hospital's management.

> The mess in my office was as reassuring to them as it was to me myself. It was a place where the pressure to make sense was so much less intense than it actually was; which after all is precisely what I wanted it to be.
>
> (Grainger, 2010: 17)

There is a quite intriguing paradox in all this: the hospital's mission seems to remove chaos from the society, putting it in a container where it can be ruled and made harmless; on the other hand, the messy beauty therapy room is like a little wild and hazy oasis in a structure striving for order, a special space where chaos can be re-admitted and tolerated.

Once the space had been established, and more and more people came to visit it, Roger started thinking about something to entertain them. He thought his acting experience might prove useful in a place where some people were actually *disturbed*, but a lot of other people were just *bored*. But he couldn't imagine how. So, for inspiration, he went to see a person who had had a huge influence on him in the past, the director and producer Joan Littlewood. On the day of his visit, the theatre was closed for shows, and Joan used to open it up to the neighbourhood kids, who could use the costumes, props and everything else, and they could go wild on stage at their liking. Joan said that they were just enjoying pretending: the children are holding a 'mucking around' session, she explained. And Roger said to himself: 'this is what I want: I want to give the people in the department the opportunity to have "mucking around" sessions'!

> The whole thing tends to be unruly, hilarious, anarchic. (…) Some of the patients take a stern view of it all, deploring the chaplain's involvement in such frivolous activities. (…) People seem to be enjoying themselves all right, but surely that is not the point. (…) The point here seems to be that people should 'know their place'. And the chaplain's place, as everybody

knows, is in the chapel, on Sundays. (…) It is certainly a bit strange to find the chaplaincy taking on a role which combines the characteristics of theatrical impresario, circus-master and buffoon. Perhaps one is in fact justified in wanting to know what all this has, in fact, got to do with religion?.

(Grainger, 1979: 96)

Finding an answer to the latter question will be the focus of Roger's inquiry for the decades to follow, as it is recorded in his books and articles spanning from the early 70s to 2013. He found himself needing to reconcile those two ostensibly incompatible roles he himself was playing, the priest and the actor, as well as reconciling Church and Theatre, which had been fierce enemies for centuries. Lastly, it entails unravelling the connections between people's therapeutic and spiritual needs, which are usually seen as excluding each other and rarely are objects of interest for academic research.

However, when I first heard the story in the cosy and warm restaurant room, carefully tasting our hot soups while the snow was storming outside, I realized that the seeds of the answer were already there, in that improbable and naïve 'mucking around experiment'. People freely and candidly playing together in the beauty therapy room were not just entertaining themselves in order to escape the boredom of institutional life. They were meeting each other in a special space where judgement was not ruling (a forgiveness space) and where they could be set free for a while from everyday concerns about themselves and their own state of suffering, looking at their fellow inmates in a new way, as playmates. Inhabiting that odd and fuzzy but clearly recognizable space, carved out against the mind-slating machinery of the hospital, they could provisionally and gently break their protective shells and allow themselves to be curious and interested in the others. This 'stretching towards' is not just a trivial event, a practical consequence of the 'rules of the game', but is the seed of relationship; it renews and revitalizes people's abilities to create bonds among each other.

Drama communicates by means of our awareness of having some kind of personal relationship with the people in the play who have been brought to life by the action of shared imagination as this becomes living flesh in the theatrical event. In the play, we recognise our fellow human beings and reach out to them in love. The play is a place where we are healed by love: a place where we can find out how love really works, perhaps even what it really is.

(Grainger, 1995: 14)

## The Intersubjective Side of Dramatherapy

This focus on relationships is what I call the intersubjective side of dramatherapy. I have elsewhere inquired about the connection between intersubjectivity and dramatherapy (Pitruzzella, 2015, 2016, 2017, 2018) and will revisit this notion in the following part of this chapter. According to the intersubjective perspective, we are born into a world of relationships, for which we are biologically disposed. Intersubjective dialogues are present in newborn babies, even before birth; they are musically oriented and occur before a notion of self appears. This innate disposition is inscribed both in our brain and in our body, and it is the basis for the development of empathy. If these hypotheses are true, we can affirm that restoring intersubjective abilities mainly consists in unearthing potentialities that are already there, even when they are concealed under layers of suffering and confusion. And dramatherapy is a helpful method to do it. What I want to maintain here is that it was implicit in Roger's intention in dramatherapy:

> It is the dramatic principle which is being explored and developed here: a way of looking at, and participating in, life which 'speaks the language' of human relationships, the language of human loving.
>
> (Grainger, 1995: 12)

And the way this dramatic principle manifests itself in our special space is through the systematic use of embodied and shared imagination.

> Imagination is really another dimension of personal and social being, one whenever I enter it releases me from my preoccupation with my own actions and intentions and sets me free to pursue the completeness I long for and do not find anywhere except in encounter with the otherness which establishes my own very separate personal identity. This is a doctrine of the imagination which allows it to perform a completely different role from that of an expression of the self - that of moving beyond itself to find a new way of being itself. The experience is not simply one of expanding the area or scope of the self, but of *leaving it behind*.
>
> (Duggan and Grainger, 1997: 18)

## The Spiritual Side of Dramatherapy

'Leaving the self behind' is the spiritual side of dramatherapy. Perhaps it could be useful at this point to define what I mean with this term 'spiritual' that I have already used several times. The word 'spiritual' finds its roots in the word 'spirit' which is usually intended, at least, in three different ways. The first is connected with some form of religious belief, in which the term 'spirit' refers to supernatural beings, like gods, angels or demons, and their manifestations. The second with some philosophical quests, which acknowledge 'spirit' as the transcendent energy moving the whole universe. The third with a traditional view of human nature as threefold: body (the physical part), mind (the reasoning part) and spirit (the most valuable part, which is eternal and connects us with some extramundane reality). The common notion of spirituality is usually related to these three ways of defining 'spirit'. My personal use of the word 'spirituality' does not exactly match any of these meanings, skipping the question of what actually 'spirit' is: I refer instead to a tendency (which is often perceived as an inner urge) to transcend the borders of the ego and the constraints of the material world, looking towards a higher level of awareness that can give a truest and profoundest meaning to life.

This is the sense I perceive in Roger's idea of drama: a place where people celebrate their mutual encounter through actively playing with their shared imagination, and in doing so, they temporally unleash themselves from the fetters and the burdens of their weighted and worried selves. And, as each one stretches towards the other, they create a space between them in which an ego-transcendent experience can manifest itself in practice. This is not a miracle: we are not expected to see God either in a dazzling whirlwind or in a burning bramble bush. Roger explained this experience in the terms of Martin Buber's dialogical philosophy. Buber had described with intense images what relationships should really be: for him, we live in a world that has two faces, corresponding to two different attitudes we have towards it. I can look at the other as an object to be inquired, assessed and judged: I pronounce what Buber calls 'the fundamental word *I-It*'. But this position barely marks the experience of the other, not yet the relationship. 'Relationship is reciprocity', says Buber; it can happen when I turn again towards the other as a subject and say the fundamental word *I-Thou*, which is at the heart of the encounter. Life oscillates between these two poles, alternating identification with the other and separation from the other, harmonized in a vital cycle: '*I-It* is the eternal chrysalis; *I-Thou* is the eternal butterfly' (Buber, 1923: 59). In this continuous shifting between the two positions, which is the rhythm of human life, Roger had envisioned the creation of a space between people, a space that at the same time divides and connects, which he called 'betweenness'.

> Value for human beings is 'in the space between', the separation which allows relationship. To try to live in 'Thou' is to be painfully limited by the experience of someone else's being, restricting one's thoughts and feelings to those learned from them. To try to live in 'It' is to forswear real personal contact, and enjoy the omnipotence of 'pure' thought unfettered by human circumstance. (...) In drama, withdrawal and encounter, courage and self-preservation oscillate to maintain a kind of relational balance of thought and experience that is genuinely human, and, according to Buber, genuinely religious (...): 'Every particular "Thou" is a glimpse through to the eternal "Thou"' [Buber, 1961: 75].
>
> (in Grainger, 1995: 25)

You may have noted the many analogies between the actions performed by the characters of the two stories, which can be epitomized in Roger's three-fold metaphor: 'Clear the space. Claim the space. Sanctify the space'. Both the characters look for a good enough place, and when they have found it, they re-arrange it in order to set it somehow apart from the surrounding space.

Once redefined as a special enclosure with clear boundaries, it is ready to be enlivened by the action of people who momentarily inhabit it, and it becomes a place where love and relationship can be cultivated. We can be sure that this place is safe enough for us to live not only because it has boundaries and rules, but mostly because it is a place where love among people becomes a mirror of a more encompassing love, which includes all beings, to whom we should not forget to bid 'Goodnight'. And this was resounding with my experience of that moment, while saying 'Thou' to the person who would be my friend and mentor for many years to come and experiencing a profound encounter that turned for a while that tiny dining room into a sanctuary.

## What is Space Made of?

Before discussing further this threefold metaphor in the last section of this chapter, showing how it can enlighten some healing factors of dramatherapy, I would like to address a pivotal question: what is space made of?

We know that at a very basic level (which has been inquired by that mind-blowing field of science called quantum physics), everything is mostly made of emptiness, and even those we can sometimes identify as concrete matter particles soon vanish in waves, parcels of energy, strings or anything fuzzy and undetermined when we try to look at them closely. Nevertheless, people's everyday experience of the world is totally different. I have a body that is fundamentally made of the same insubstantial substance of which the rest of the world is composed (and maybe the same stuff as dreams are made on), and I move it in a material world that is basically as inconsistent as it is. In my everyday experience, however, I perceive my body as a solid matter: with some effort, I can move it to my liking and use it to interact with other material bodies and objects. Between my body and them, there is something I call space. Whether this space is totally void or occupied by some invisible things like ether or a wisely mixed blend of oxygen and other gases (made by particles that, in their turn, are nothing more than small bundles of energy floating in the unescapable emptiness), it does not really matter at this level until I can cross it to come closer to the other bodies and objects.

From a subjective point of view, however, space is not just a neutral medium to be crossed when necessary; it has been clearly shown that each of us perceives the space immediately around his or her body as highly significant. In the early eighties, Giacomo Rizzolatti put forward the concept of 'peripersonal space', by identifying a set of motor neurons that responded to events occurring in the immediate area around people's bodies as if they were occurring *to* their body (Rizzolatti *et al.*, 1981). In further researches, peripersonal space has been defined as a 'multisensory-motor interface between the individual and the environment; (…) a spatial extension of the body, playing a key role in defensive and approaching behaviour' (Noel *et al.*, 2021: 25). Michael S. A. Graziano (2018) maintains that this neural arrangement evolved as a protective tool, allowing our ancestors to discern instantaneously any immediate threats to their bodies, especially the most sensitive parts, like the face, the head and the upper arms. It was already known, at least since Penfield's *homunculus,* that the senso-motor neurons encoding these body parts in the brain are more extended and active than the other; what is remarkable is that this encoding involves also the space surrounding them, as well as the rest of the body, albeit to a lesser extent. Researchers point to the fact that, by virtue of the brain's plasticity, peripersonal space is rather dynamic: it can broaden to include tools we use with our hands (think about handling your phone ...) (Cléry *et al.,* 2015); it can shrink or expand according to our mood (De Vignemont and Iannetti, 2014); it can be enlarged as to include other people in it (Coello and Iachini, 2021). So, the space that we perceive as an extension of our body can be a protective armour, a border against invasion, but it can be also a welcoming space.

Our bodies are in space, so the space we perceive must have a fundamental physical quality. But it is likewise true that most of the time we define space by endowing it with a meaning, which is an exquisitely mental operation. In a similar way that my biologically founded peripersonal space can have at the same time a defensive and a bonding function, my room can be either a place where I feel free and comfortable, to the point of leaving the door open for friends coming, or a secured and closed space in order to defend myself from the outside world, or even a mix of the two. Materially speaking, my body is still my body, in a room whose walls and furniture are the same, but they are in fact two totally different spaces. We cannot deny that space is mostly a mental concept.

What then? People who had read my previous works know that my position on the body–mind issue is informed by the non-dualistic philosophic stance of Baruch Spinoza. The Dutch philosopher came to confute the model of Descartes, who considered mind and matter (the latter including our physical body) as two different and opposing substances: *Res cogitans* (thinking thing) and *Res extensa* (extended thing). Accordingly, the mind is an incorporeal principle that, by God's grace, is able to govern and guide the body more or less than as we drive our cars. This is not actually a metaphor that Descartes could have used, but it is quite in line with the way this body/mind model has been interpreted in the following centuries, up to Gilbert Ryle's striking image of 'the ghost in the machine'. Spinoza rejects this dualism asserting that if a substance exists, it cannot be but one. What might seem to be different things are merely different ways in which one substance exists. God is Nature, and Nature is God, the one and only substance, infinite and eternal: *Deus sive Natura.* Although we cannot transcend our finite condition, we can none-theless partake in the infinite and eternal substance of God/Nature, as we share some of the infinite attributes through which it manifests itself in the finite modes of the finite world. These attributes are Thought and Extension, which, in human experience, are perceived as mind and body. They are the modes of our existence in the world, but they are essential aspects of the one and only substance. As an undivided part of the whole Nature, this unity, which is the human being itself, is subjected to the same laws that rule Nature, which we can be able to recognize and comprehend.

Space is at the same time in our minds and around our bodies, but we could definitely say the contrary: space is in our bodies and around our minds. I maintain that the notion of space cannot be comprehended unless under the light of a non-dualistic perspective, in which body and mind are just accounts of the same phenomenon from different points of view. This perspective implies that whatever happens in our bodies, happens in our minds and vice-versa. And this is exactly how drama works.

## Dramatic Space

The ghastly fratricidal founding myth of the Roman Empire tells us of Romulus, one of the twin wolf-bred brothers, who wants to be king of the future city, digging a long ditch to set up the walls; when his brother Remus crosses the ditch, Romulus slaughters him. This myth is maybe echoing the great change in people's relationship with the environment marked by the Neolithic agricultural revolution and the consequential birth of land ownership, which was nonsense for the old hunter-gatherer tribes who had roamed the Earth for many millennia. As people ceased to be nomads and needed a lasting place to cultivate the land and breeding livestock, it was necessary to make clear that that particular space belonged to them and to no one else, and that they were eager to protect it at all costs. Even if here and there few traces of violent acts have been found all along the Palaeolithic period, the earliest evidence of actual warfare dates around 7.500 BC, when the new economy that eventually will produce cities and empires had been already set, although in a small scale. Jean-Jacques Rousseau made clear statements on all this: 'the first person who, having enclosed a plot of land, took it into his head to say this is mine and found people simple enough to believe him, was the true founder of civil society. What crimes, wars, murders, miseries and horrors would the human race have been spared had someone pulled up the stakes or filled in the ditch and cried out to his fellow men: do not listen to this imposter. You are lost if you forget that the fruits of the earth belong to all and the earth to no one!' (Rousseau, 1762: 207). Making boundaries can be an arbitrary and violent act; by drawing a line, I arrogate for myself the right to decide who is in and who is out, and consequentially, who is right and who is wrong, and who is good and who is bad. The space-creating tendency we have inherited from our Neolithic ancestors looks really like a curse.

Yet there is also another side of this tendency, which acts in a contrary way and creates spaces not for exclusion but for inclusion. This is the clearing of the sacred space. Roger did not deny that the primal gesture of marking boundaries to create space is at least ambivalent, having an implicit defensive and aggressive value. However, since the dawn of time, people have also created spaces to gather together and let the numinous manifest itself. And, as Roger maintained, what really matters is not the tangible quality of the place we identify as a sacred space, but the meaning we ascribe to it.

> Sacred space (...) can be induced or created quite simply in all sorts of places. The most important thing, however, is the intention to draw near to sacredness, and the action of setting space and time apart in order to do so.
>
> (Grainger, 2014: 79)

As we have seen, in Roger's vision, the process that establishes drama is substantially analogous to the setting of a sacred space: 'Clear the space' means setting the stage for the dramatic experience to occur; 'Claim the space' means actively inhabiting the stage, letting ourselves entirely be into the experience; 'Sanctify the space' is handling the stage, celebrating the shared experience, and thus renovating the stage as a place where the fundamental word 'I-Thou' can be pronounced:

> Space itself is the archetype, because it symbolises an expectant absence, a possibility of ultimate encounter, the meaning beyond any kind of appearance. (...) The empty space is the total archetype of transcendence because it presents us with infinite possibility. (...) It is dramatic space, therapeutic space, sacred space.
>
> (Grainger, 2014: 86)

Roger Grainger died in September 2015, his car being swamped by an anomalous wave while crossing the bridge between the mainland and the small Achill Island, which was his last residence. I had the news the same day I was supposed to run a dramatherapy masterclass at the ECArTE Conference in Palermo, whose title was *Beyond identities: the intersubjective dimension of dramatherapy* and was largely based on Roger's ideas. I was overwhelmed by grief, and my first reaction was to cancel the masterclass; however, with the warm support of friends and colleagues, I eventually decided to do it anyway, intentionally devoting it to celebrate Roger's legacy. So, we cleared the space and then we claimed it, and when eventually we sanctified it, when the bliss of betweenness was glaring among people, it was clear for everybody that he was there, 'mucking around' with us, and I had the feeling that he will be with me every time a space opens for betweenness to occur. And it actually happened; but this is another story, which I will tell you another time ...

## References

Buber, M. (1923) *Il Principio Dialogico*. Milano: San Paolo, p. 1993.

Cléry, J., et al. (2015) 'Neuronal bases of peripersonal and extrapersonal spaces, their plasticity and their dynamics: Knowns and unknowns', *Neuropsychologia*, 70, pp. 313–326.

Coello, Y. and Iachini, T. (2021) 'The Social Dimension of Peripersonal Space', in De Vignemont, F., et al. (ed.) *The World at Our Fingertips*. Oxford: Oxford University Press, pp. 267–284.

De Angulo, J. (1953) *Indian Tales*. New York: North Point Press.

De Vignemont, F. and Iannetti, G.D. (2014) 'How many peripersonal spaces?' *Neuropsychologia*. 10.1016/j.neuropsychologia.2014.11.018

Duggan, M. and Grainger, R. (1997) *Imagination, Identification and Catharsis in Theatre and Therapy*. London: Jessica Kingsley.

Grainger, R. (1979) *Watching for Wings. Theology and Mental Illness in a Pastoral Setting*. London: Darton, Longman & Todd.

Grainger, R. (1995) *The Glass of Heaven. The Faith of the Dramatherapist*. London: Jessica Kingsley.

Grainger, R. (2010) 'Can anybody tell me who I am? A memory of institutional dramatherapy', *Dramatherapy*, 32(1), pp. 17–20.

Grainger, R. (2010) *Suspending Disbelief. Theatre as Context for Sharing*. Brighton: Sussex Academic Press.

Grainger, R. (2014) *Ritual and Theatre*. London: Austin Macauley Publisher.

Graziano, M.S.A. (2018) *The Spaces Between Us: A Story of Neuroscience, Evolution, and Human Nature*. New York: Oxford University Press.

Noel, N.-P., et al. (2021) 'Peri-Personal Space as an Interface for Self-Environment Interaction', in De Vignemont, F., et al. (ed.) *The World at Our Fingertips*. Oxford: Oxford University Press, pp. 18–46.

Pitruzzella, S. (2015) 'In Search of the Lost Mirror. Dramatherapy, Intersubjectivity and the Autistic Spectrum', in Hougham, R., Pitruzzella, S. and Scoble, S., (eds.) *Dimensions of Reflection in the Arts Therapies*. Plymouth: Plymouth University Press.

Pitruzzella, S. (2016) *Drama, Creativity and Intersubjectivity: Foundations of Change in Dramatherapy*. London: Routledge.

Pitruzzella, S. (2017) 'The Intersubjective Dimension of Dramatherapy', in Hougham, R., Pitruzzella, S. and Scoble, S. (eds.) *Cultural Landscapes in the Arts Therapies*. Plymouth: Plymouth University Press.

Pitruzzella, S. (2018) 'The space that divides and connects. Betweenness and the intersubjective perspective', *Dramatherapy*, 39(1), p. 2018.

Rizzolatti, G., Scandolara, C., Matelli, M. and Gentilucci, M. (1981) 'Afferent properties of periarcuate neurons in macaque monkeys. II. Visual responses', *Behavioural Brain Research*, 2(2), pp. 147–163.

Rousseau, J.J. (1762) *The Social Contract and Discourses by Jean-Jacques Rousseau*, translated with an Introduction by Cole, G.D.H., London & Toronto: J.M. Dent and Sons, p. 1923.

# 10 Liminality and Ritual in Dramatherapy – The Intersubjective Space

*Joanna Jaaniste*

This chapter considers the intersubjective space and what it means when observed alongside ritual and liminality. Peter Brook calls the space 'a bare stage', continuing as follows: 'a man walks across this empty space whilst someone else is watching him, and this is all that is needed for an act of theatre to be engaged' (Brook, 2008: 11). For Brook, in this space, theatre is engaged in the meeting of two people, which sparks drama. Drama, from the Greek *dran*, means 'to do', calling to mind this *act* or *action*. The act or deed of the person (actor) who walks the stage space is a ritual act, and the witness is their audience; intersubjectivity produces the drama.

Dramatherapist Phil Jones, as well as devoting many pages to the play space, gives a definition of drama as opposed to theatre, based mainly on Landy's understanding of drama as 'a separation of self and non-self ... a separation of realities' (1982: 21). Jones defines drama as 'an entry into a special state where individuals, the space they use and the things they do, exist in a pretended reality' (1996: 13). This *special state* can be connected with liminality, in which the transitional liminal space can be understood as beyond the personal and encompassing a new threshold of consciousness (Roose-Evans, 1994). This chapter includes vignettes of dramatherapy sessions illustrating the concept of space through the lenses of liminality and ritual.

## The *Active Absence* of Space

David Read Johnson (2010) says that 'Theatre, like poetry, gives room for gaps, empty spaces that give rise to the shadows unseen in conversation and prose' (2010: 62). Bortoft sees actors as using their role as a point of entry to the stage. They encounter the space as an 'active absence' which starts to move them. Then they start to be 'acted by the play' instead of trying to act the play (Bortoft, 2018: 15). The intersubjectivity rests on this concept when there is more than one person on stage. Bachelard, in *The Poetics of Space* (2014), writes fulsomely about homes and buildings filled with invisible poetry before anyone walks into them. Bachelard writes of the memory of a warm space where one has once lived that does not call out to be expanded, but wants to be dwelt within. The later life version of the inhabitant's

DOI: 10.4324/9781003252399-14

warm-space memory, he considers, can change its shape, temperature and size to become the stuff of daydreams. Bachelard's strong link with the poetic imagination reminds me of Shakespeare's line from A Midsummer Night's Dream, where the poet's pen and their imagination 'gives to airy nothing/A place of habitation and a name' (Shakespeare, 2007: A Midsummer Night's Dream, V. 1.16–1.17). This invisibility and dream space exist however in a concrete dimension. So, what of the stage before the actor walks across it? The architectural critic Gray Read (2005), in his commentary on the 1930s establishment of the Theatre of Space in Paris, says:

> Every room is a stage, every public space is a theatre, and every façade is a backdrop. Each has places for entry and exit, scenery, props, and a design that sets up potential relationships between people. In this sense, architecture and theatre are sister arts, creating worlds where people interact in studied spatial relationships. (2005: 33)

Elsewhere, Read (2013) sees Brook's work as architectural, building an ambience where the imagination of the cast on stage can come alive. He also argues as an architectural critic that once there is an audience, the so-called empty stage expands and becomes activated, 'press[ing] into the fullness of the city to make a place for thought and action' (2013: 4). His view approaches my own personally lived belief that thought-forms exist in certain spaces, along with silent echoes of words spoken there in earlier times.

On a personal note, as a 19-year-old in my first job in London's Soho, I had to walk past several strip clubs on my way to work and going home. I sensed the echoes of the people, workers and audience members who over many years had anticipatory thoughts on entering and reflections on exiting through their doors. I compared myself to a concept of the very different sensing experience of centuries of prayer and meditation on entering a building like Westminster Abbey, imagining myself wearing a blindfold to do so. I decided that although the dank smell and lack of warmth therein could be telling factors on entry, there was definitely a contrasting *active absence* in each case. I argue that whatever space we see our clients in, it is important to notice and be aware of what it already holds before we entered it. It may influence our ritual and inspire liminality.

## The Concept of Space in the Practice of Dramatherapy

In a reading of dramatherapy literature, I have found that there is a significantly higher ratio of references to ritual in comparison with the space or place where it happens, although we can gain some clues about the nature of space from the architectural corpus. In searching the literature where the word 'space' appears in the title of contributions, I came across Pitruzella's (2018) writing on the topic of intersubjectivity and the 'space that divides and connects' (Pitruzella, 2018: 3). He writes about the late Roger Grainger, his close colleague, whose books and expertise as a dramatherapist encouraged him to think about Buber's I-Thou and I-It theories, and the intersubjective and interactive spaces that lie between them. He explains how Grainger's own exemplary skill with participants brought relational warmth into the dramatherapy space. I resonated with this, since Roger was the person who inspired me to take up the dramatherapy training I had been offered 30 years ago following five 3-hour sessions that he gave at the Dramatherapy North conference in Manchester in 1992. Both my recollection of those workshops and Pitruzella's experience of Roger's session for students reminded me that the space can either divide or connect – an important concept in considering ritual. It seems that in both cases, there was a memorable sensibility of intersubjective connection between the presenter and participants. The impression of liminality that is possible through the *between-ness* that Pitruzella later describes as *spiritual magic* (2018: 7–8) was certainly there for me in that Manchester University tutorial room space. From my recollection, each person had experienced something meaningful, and my own interconnection with the poem 'Kangaroo' by D.H. Lawrence (1994: 322), brought by Roger, was a liminal reminder of my adopted homeland of Australia and place of choice, far away.

Chesners' more practical advice about space is also helpful, especially for dramatherapists working in spaces where one might be interrupted. She writes about safety for the client and the need for a protective space at a regular meeting time (1994: 59). This framing for the sessions is important, as the dramatherapy space should be private and free from disturbance, as Roger's was, a place where clients can be sure of confidentiality as well as physical, psychological and emotional safety. Dramatherapy vignettes in this chapter take place in spaces where these important requirements cannot be overlooked and where the active absence must also be acknowledged.

## Space and Ritual in Dramatherapy

Winnicott encourages us to pay attention to our environment, which he saw as spreading out into a creative and elevated sense of the being of humanity: 'I have located this important area of experience in the potential space between the individual and the environment ... [a space] which both joins and separates' (Winnicott, 1994: 102–103). Winnicott's interpersonal joining and separation in the transitional space, with its origins in the original distance between mother and infant, has everything to do with ritual. It echoes the work done by Grainger (1990; 1995) and Pitruzella (2018) and isolates the space where the inner self and the environment meet and where the drama takes place intersubjectively. Young children have a natural consciousness of it. Their creative translation of life events through play and ritual are the beginnings of what Turner (1967) and van Gennep (1960) considered essential for rites of passage leading into adulthood in a healthy way.

The early dramatherapy pioneers saw a connection between ritual and rites of passage (in Shamanism, in tribal cultures, in the theatre) and dramatherapy practice. Peter Slade (1954), in his publication *Child Drama,* alludes to the idea that a community which has not lost its rituals enjoys better mental health than one where everyone is a subjective spectator. In ritual there is performance, and in performance there is both actor and witness. The young child who witnesses their caregiver in daily life often takes on these roles through imitation. A child who has imitated their caregivers has a better chance of developing well than those who have not (Schrier, 2014).

An essential part of human development affords children the power of imitation to use objects and perform with others. Children's inner memories of events are transformed into important life happenings so that they can make sense of them. They are connected with the metaphor and magical substance of the space of the environment where the memories came into being (Mussa, 2016).

For people of any age in dramatherapy, the creative exploration of life stages requires that the dramatherapist offers a secure space for vulnerability (past, present or both) to be engaged with, both verbally or physically. As is well-known and understood by dramatherapists, drama does not need words. Lawson (2001) believes that during our lives, humans may, to a greater extent, interconnect physically through space than with words. He observes that when we walk into a space, other people read our 'spatial language' long before we say anything at all (2001: 2). This phenomenon is commonly known as body language. Sue Jennings (1973) makes the point that in the Western spectator-based society, moving the body in space, especially in a group, enables people to discover and share new forms of ritual. This observation has gathered more significance since it was written nearly half a century ago; we now share screens and rely ever more on individual work than interacting in groups, especially in the era of Covid-19 with all its variants. Even on screen, the existing magic engendered through time in the space we are occupying can assist the ritual to evolve. In dramatherapy groups online, ritualized intersubjective mirroring is possible. In the therapeutic exchange, this can happen through embodiment.

Ritual encompasses rites of passage that a secular society often overlooks and sometimes loses completely. In Australian cities, for example, planned for the most part by people from the other side of the world, steel and glass shopping malls have, for the most part, replaced the Eurocentric fountains and sculptures they were familiar with that can be markers and reminders of these rites. Grainger (1995), not only a dramatherapist but also a pastor, brought his theological wisdom to bear on the sacred connections available to the dramatherapy practitioner offering the ritual. He believed that biblical word pictures, which refer to death and resurrection, can give us an important grounding, even in a secular society, for dealing with death and other changes taking place in our lives. His writing refers to the suspension of time in sacred stories and events which, for example, can give people with serious issues such as responses to complex trauma or serious illness in their lives a new way of reframing their journey, of seeing the world, and their place in it: 'because of their reference to infinity, rites of passage are ways of restoring us to our original identity. They reconcile the primal to whatever is to come, allowing us to experience a life renewed and full of possibility' (Grainger, 1995: 57).

We can also find these rituals expressed in fairy tales, where the overlooked youngest child is given challenges to perform before inner transformation can take place in their environment. Once the tasks are completed, they can return to their community, offering the wisdom of their encounters. Van Gennep (1960) defines these stages as separation, transition and homecoming. So many ancient tales, with their broad narrative landscapes, give us the space to work with ritual, and Grainger gives us a way of approaching the narratives as healing events, transformative in the way they combine with the therapeutic power of drama (Grainger, 1995).

## Liminality

Liminality has evolved from the word 'limen', which means a threshold, doorway or crossing place. Turner (1982) extended this concept, interpreting liminality as a series of separate hallowed spaces, an idea which was developed by Holmwood and Scales (2018). Van Gennep's three stages (1960) of rites of passage are doorways to pass through: the childhood separation from family, initiation into adulthood and then acceptance into adult society. Holmwood proposes an argument for a liminal space between each stage, identifying the 'between-ness' of liminality and doors within doors. El Wardany (2020) writes about humans waking from a metaphysical sleep, freedom only dawning upon them if they invoke the fragmented past so that it might be revitalized by the present moment, altering the relationship between past and present. This concept has relevance for the liminal space which greets dramatherapy participants when they enter the play space with its *active absence*. The human soul needs a space whose symbolic sacredness can be woken up to, in all its transitional or archetypal resonance.

The theatre stage has had many incarnations of sacredness throughout history, as Pendzik (1994) has documented in some detail. She takes the reader through the long and poignant relationship between the stage and the shared mystical space and its significance from the point of view of therapy. Ancient shamanistic rituals have many links with theatre, as do the boat journeys of the pharaohs into the afterlife and the circular space around altars to Dionysus in Greece. On my visit to Epidavros a few years ago, I could barely tear myself away from the herb-scented grassy area between the famous amphitheatre and the ruins of the Aesculapian temple. The scene intensified for me the connection between theatre and medicine, Asclepius being the Greek god of healing. I could picture families taking their unwell members to see the play and witness its renewing properties in the Dionysian festivals of old. The space had echoes of the tragedy absorbed by the minds of the audience members and the catharsis experienced in their bodies (Halliwell and Aristotle, 1998).

Pendzik (1994) writes about many styles of stage and architectural arrangements, from the *axis mundi* or central column, believed in Northern Europe to hold up the world, to the proscenium arch of Elizabethan times and beyond. She pauses in the first third of the twentieth century, when all structure disappeared, which was seen by some as a rejection of the sacred space of theatre. Pendzik (1994) quotes Artaud, who regarded this dematerialization of the space as a restoration of the unbroken connection between the actor and the audience. In this space, Artaud encapsulates the twentieth-century path towards the spectator becoming more readily enfolded in the action and more deeply affected by its proximity. Pendzik sees this as a return to a time when the stage was actually an aspect of the sacred space and the central locus relating to the four cardinal directions, referencing the Dionysian altar or the central pillar of the shaman's abode.

The liminality that exists in the dramatherapy space is available to both the dramatherapist and the client. The separation that both Turner (1982) and van Gennep (1960) suggest, an important characteristic of liminality, is key to the creative space. Participants in the drama can separate themselves from the world of routine, the formalities of keeping records and the everydayness of life. 'For me, the essence of liminality is to be found in its release from normal constraints, making possible the deconstruction of the "uninteresting" constructions of common sense, the meaningfulness of ordinary life' (Turner, 1977: 68).

Atalandi Apergi (2014) finds in her multi-cultural work as a dramatherapist in Greece that for refugees and immigrants, 'there are often no rituals to mark the loss of way of life, home, identity, connection with a community and culture' (2014: 125), and that dramatherapy can provide such rituals. She refers to Turner's (1995) view of liminality where a participant's identification with self can become somewhat mysterious, resulting in some blurring, but also presenting an opportunity for space to expand, allowing the participant to come home to self in a different way. Like her, I find the space is available wherever I work, but particularly in my own studio, to offer an entry point for liminality.

---

**Vignette 1 – The threshold**

The small studio, in the garden of my home, was architect-designed and purpose built for dramatherapy and completed in 2000. At the time of working with the client described in this vignette, I had offered individual sessions there for 15 years. The space had therefore evolved and matured somewhat and had the active absence of the work with past clients from many cultures. It had even once served as a refuge for an Indonesian client with identity dissociative disorder. On one occasion when I was not there, her 'three-year-old self' had wandered from her home and through my unlocked garden gate without my prior knowledge and I had to be called back home to assure her that only her adult self was permitted to make an appointment to see me. Ever since then, it has had a stronger personal meaning for me as a sanctuary for clients.

Selina, a 22-year-old woman, was a citizen of the United Kingdom who had come to Australia on a working holiday visa, and with a few weeks remaining before she returned home, she consulted me for dramatherapy. She told me straight away that she wanted to be more 'self-aware' and 'out there'. In the first session, she revealed her place in the family within its constellation, by grouping together the inner members of a babushka doll, with a figure for each person. Selina's doll was the largest after her mum's and stepfather's, but it was squashed behind their dolls and tightly squeezed between her sister's and her dad's.

In our second session, I spent an hour playing with Selina. She moved around as we brandished, wore or curled up in coloured cloths. Her breathing tended to be shallow, even though she had studied drama at university, and I put this down to shyness. She chose black and I chose yellow. Selina tried to push me into a corner of the space without much eye contact. I felt squashed, rather like her doll. I wondered why, asking if there was anyone she wished to push away? It turned out to be her manager at the café where she worked, who Selina said was a 'bitch', because she was criticizing Selina's work when she was 'just trying to do [her] job'. I thought Selina was 'out there' already, in the sense of seeking adventure on the other side of the world, although not in the sense of feeling confident to stand up to the manager at the time. I encouraged her to use 'I' rather than 'you' as she spoke about her experiences.

In the following session, we worked with projective objects and Selina chose an aeroplane and a photo of a group of children from a collection of toys and images. Projection is a technique used to externalize a participant's issue so that by distancing them in this way, they can understand the problem in a new way. Using their imaginations, clients project attributes of themselves into scarves or other props used on stage and in the theatre. Reversing roles with the aeroplane, she stamped and called to it as she marched towards the door, seeming to say, 'you just watch me!' At our moment of reflection, she said of that enactment: 'I was pushing myself towards awareness'. She told me that she had always had a happy life, without the kinds of problems that can bring opportunities for self-understanding. The photograph brought up a memory of bullying – not of herself, as she had always been the kind of child who would tell the boys off and support the victim – 'not at 13 though'. I had a picture of a child who was popular and spoke her mind at school, and with puberty, that chutzpah went into retirement while she developed into an adult. I remembered my own experience of being bullied – asking my parents if I could change my name as a child because of a bullying chant including my name directed at me. I shared this with her, and we spoke about the importance of names.

In Selina's fourth session, she chose a fairy tale to perform: *Rumpelstiltskin*. She wanted to be the miller's daughter and I took on the other roles. I asked her how she felt in the story's dramatization when she had nothing more to give the little man, who wanted a reward for helping her spin straw into gold. She said, 'I was *heartbroken*'. The emphasis she gave this word stood out for me. In reflection at the end of the session, Selina was able to say that her character's final treatment of the little man, where she tells him his name, was justified and this helped her realize that she could have spoken more firmly to her manager at the café. Selina was very comfortable with her role and the fairy tale – it seemed as though this was her milieu. The 'naming' had reappeared in our work. There was a sense of liminality for me then, as there had been when she had gone towards the door in the third session; she wanted to be 'out there', on the other side of that threshold, and have her 'name' spoken and heard.

The following week, Selina came to the session feeling disturbed because a shocking memory had come back to her. She had written in a journal after each session, and this had helped her to identify a time when she had been heartbroken in her life. A close relative, an aunt, had been murdered when she was ten years old. A great deal of this session was spent in grieving, as she had blocked out this memory for many years and no one in the family had spoken of it since. I told her a story of death, grief and transformation: *Ulu and the breadfruit tree* (Gersie and King, 1990) which I have found helpful in grieving sessions with others. She drew a picture of a series of breadfruit trees at different stages of maturity, which I recognized as markers of her own rites of passage. As she had not been able to attend the relative's funeral since it took place in the USA where the aunt lived, I asked her if she would like to use the sixth session to celebrate her aunt's life, and she agreed.

In this important penultimate session, Selina was able to enter into a role reversal with her lost loved one and say goodbye, describing what her aunt had meant to her during her life. She had brought the dead woman's well-loved music, and we decorated the room with yellow flowers and cloths – it had been her favourite colour. Selina said that she would open up later about this tragedy to her family, especially to her mother, and this would make them both feel stronger. For both of us, the little studio seemed to expand into a very different space filled with light which belonged to her aunt, wherever she was in an afterlife, like Read's (2013) intersubjective special expansion once there is an actor and a witness.

Selina's very last session was spent enacting some of the earlier work as a celebration of our time together. We moved around again with cloths, and the play was very different this time – much more cooperative and fun. Selina's breathing was more regular, and her eye contact with me was very clear. At the end, when I asked her what she was taking away from our work, she said, 'Dramatherapy is an eye-opener'. The session ended in laughter, as we both realized the implications of 'I-opener'.

She felt she was on her way to achieving her self-awareness goal as she walked through the door for the last time; the liminal inside space had encouraged her to be 'out there'.

## Play

The human imagination enables us to dream up alternative realities, and most children have a strong ability to do this, little knowing that its early practice underlies much worthwhile adult cognitive ability and reasoning. As suggested earlier, the play space is a liminal area which is important for children and adults alike. Jennings (1999) points out that the therapist, in the play space for children, must neither totally direct the play (thus deadening the forces of the child's imagination) nor abandon the child entirely to their own play devices. The latter choice leaves the child with no boundaries, which can be a very unsafe situation.

Johnson's (1986, 2005) developmental transformations (DvT) in the play space rely on the 'between-ness' that derives from a ritual structure all the way from *surface play* to *deep play*, mimicking human development. DvT is a practice which calls for the spontaneous transposing of embodied engagements in a designated playspace (Johnson, 2005). He shows how people with dementia using the *Magic Box* (an imaginary box stored in the ceiling that can be 'pulled down' and entered into through an 'as if' curtain) can structure and project concepts and ideas into it. They can then unpack some of the metaphors within the magic space, discovering and owning some of the transformations and metaphors in the process for themselves, in a different form and in a more social and conscious way (1986: 32). For elderly people with dementia, the contributions they bring to the space initially are what Johnson calls their 'surface' aspects (in other words, their appearance, age, race and shared knowledge). Even if the play comes from the surface, it is by no means superficial, as significant experiences, sensations and concerns may come to the fore at this stage. Once they have been working together for some weeks, however, deeper elements of their lives enter the play space, often manifesting through metaphor. At this stage of the play, we can see that there is more interpersonal trust, bringing about 'persona play', exploring the Self, various roles and relational involvement with family members and others (Johnson, 2005).

## Vignette 2 – Elderly participants with dementia in the play space

This group session was the final, celebratory one in a series of 16 dramatherapy sessions which took place as part of the fieldwork for my doctorate at a day centre for the elderly. In a two-arm study, participants with a diagnosis of dementia were offered dramatherapy while a second group in a day centre in Newcastle, New South Wales, engaged in usual activities (Jaaniste, 2013). During the course of the 16 weeks, the dramatherapy group had already engaged in DvT twice before and this session marked the ending of the programme. The room designated for our sessions at the day centre was usually dedicated to group meetings with clients. The staff had obviously given some thought to making the space familiar for older clients, even though some of them may not have favoured the style. It was furnished with pictures, objects and furniture from the 1940s and 50s, so we were all reminded of domestic traditions of that time and those who might have gone before us in the space. Two art therapy students and two staff members from the centre assisted with the group sessions for assessment and video recording.

Before forming the ritual of the *Magic Box*, the group greeted one another and reflected on the previous week's work. They then played with orange and black coloured silk cloths, with the contrast between the coloured cloths being remarked upon by two participants as 'our two sides', and identified by one other participant as the two sides of a human being. The group also played ball games, one of which involved throwing a word accompanying the ball to another partici-pant. Some of the words were as follows: *play, solo, grateful, silly games, company, happiness, thank you, singing* and *shared space*. They were then prepared to create and install the presence of the 'as if' imaginary circular curtain stored in the ceiling which created the Magic Box. The participants pulled it down, stepped inside and took imaginary objects from the Box.

I began by acknowledging that there were some 'mysterious things inside' the Magic Box, to which Ben (73) replied, 'There usually are'. A staff member found crystals in her imaginary box, which she handed out to the participants and Ben said, ' ... all sorts of things, up around the mountains, and all that sort of stuff, which are these things'. It seemed that Ben, whose moderate dementia was sliding into a more severe version, was offering us a metaphor for the mountains the group had climbed and the beauty of crystals found hidden in rocks. As someone who had started the programme physically rooted to the spot (like the mountain with many treasures to be found there) and 'talking about talking rather than connecting with his own feeling life' (Jaaniste, 2016: 268), he was showing us more of himself through metaphor, despite his declining health.

I asked the group if they felt as though they had climbed mountains. In answer, one of the art therapy students found some imaginary sludge – described as very viscous and green, and this got thrown around for a while, its sticky, gluey substance being examined. It came with an alarm from Neil (61): 'warning, warning!', potentially reminding us to consider the murky unfinished business that can get left to the end of a programme. Neil, by contrast, found a tree of memories growing out of the floor. The fact that it was not in the box itself, but instead coming out of the ground was significant; the tree was rooted to the floor of the therapy space and thus had something to hold on to, despite the 'unfinished business' that was sticky, formless and gel-like. Ben wanted to chop some of the tree and take it with him, so I told him that that sounded very definite. He replied, 'Yeah, and what's more, the amazing stuff around here is worth having and getting something for it. ... It sort of works, that's for sure'. The tree reminded others of twigs they had used in an earlier session, remembering the buds growing on them, signifying that there was still the presence of growth. David (74) found a bag filled with friendship rings which he proceeded to distribute to everyone. Ben found a prescription which he said he would give to his doctor and when asked what would be written on it, Ben was not sure. Neil said the doctor should be at the appointment when he'd promised and not forget to see him. David said he didn't want to see the doctor anymore and he wanted to enjoy his life. An art therapy student went on to suggest fairy cakes for the doctor and then Ben found his voice again: 'so I'll tell him a few things about this place. This – it's a good – it's a good place, actually. Down here's amazing'.

At the end of our group DvT experience, we stepped outside the curtain again and lifted it to the ceiling. After this, participants were able to choose some actual (non-imaginary) fruits and flowers to bring the programme to a close, and we sang 'We'll meet again' (Parker and Charles, 1939). The ritualized sequence in the *Magic Box* had allowed a meaningful ending to take place, with participants sharing an awareness of what they were taking away from the programme. It was interesting that the ever-increasing medicalization of dementia had also been debunked by Ben's, Neil's and David's advice to the doctor and their disregard for medical help. The process had clearly shown a preference for ritual and liminal treatment of dealing with issues and endings over some mainstream clinical treatments.

## Conclusion

Dramatherapy with individuals and groups presents the therapist and the participant(s) with an opportunity to enter a liminal space. Both parties need to be ready to meet the space they are in and to admit the unknown into the space, like the person in D.H. Lawrence's (1994: 195) poem 'The song of the man who has come through'. The protagonist of the poem says it's not so much about one's own individuality, but the breath of the spirit that blows through them.

Like the protagonist, who is warned of three dark angels who knock at the threshold in Lawrence's poem, the dramatherapist and the participant need to be available to the space and what it is telling them of its boundaries, real as a closed door or imaginary like the pull-down curtain. As Gray Read (2005) states, the entry and exit, the objects, props and design all play roles in the relational, interpersonal space where they are working. The entry into that space, the ritual which opens the therapy, the warmups, action, reflection on the work and the ending define the liminal experience that occurs.

This *special state* (Jones, 1996: 13) works intersubjectively between client and therapist and makes therapy and reflection possible. Before leaving the space, the ritualization of the ending brings the session to a close. It is then up to both professional and client, in different ways, to carry the learning that this unique state provides, transforming it to inform their ongoing journeys.

## References

Apergi, A. (2014) 'Working with liminality: A dramatherapeutic intervention with immigrants in a day care centre in Greece', *Dramatherapy*, 36(2–3), pp. 121–134.

Bortoft, H. (2018) *The Wholeness of Nature: Goethe's Way of Science*, Edinburgh: Lindisfarne Press and Floris Books.

Brook, P. (2008) *The Empty Space*. London: Penguin.

Chesner, A. (1994) 'An Integrated Model of Dramatherapy and Its Application with Adults with Learning Disabilities', in Jennings, S., Cattanach, A., Mitchell, S., Chesner, A. and Meldrum, B. (eds.) *The Handbook of Dramatherapy*. London: Routledge, pp. 58–74.

El Wardany, H. (2020) 'When waking begins'. *The Paris Review*, November 3, 2020, Big Sandy, TX. Retrieved May 25, 2020 from https://www.theparisreview.org:blog/2020/11/03/when-waking-begins/

Gersie, A. and King, N. (1990) *Storymaking in Education and Therapy*. London: Jessica Kingsley.

Grainger, R. (1990) *Drama and Healing*. London: Jessica Kingsley Publishers.

Grainger, R. (1995) *The Glass of Heaven: The Faith of the Dramatherapist*. London: Jessica Kingsley Publishers.

Halliwell, S. and Aristotle. (1998) *Aristotle's Poetics*. Chicago: University of Chicago Press.

Holmwood, C. and Scales, P. (2018) 'Liminality in Higher Education: Gaps and Moments of Uncertainty as Legitimate Learning Spaces', in Taylor, J. and Holmwood, C. (eds.) *Learning As a Creative and Developmental Process in Higher Education: A Therapeutic Arts Approach and Its Wider Application*. ProQuest E-book Central, pp. 61–71.

Jaaniste, E.J. (2013) *Pulled Through a Hedge Backwards: Improving the Quality of Life of People with Dementia Through Dramatherapy*, PhD Thesis: University of Western Sydney.

Jaaniste, J. (2016) 'Lifestage and Human Development in Dramatherapy with People Who Have Dementia', in Holmwood, C. and Jennings, S. (eds.) *Routledge International Handbook of Dramatherapy*. London & New York: Routledge, pp. 262–272.

Jennings, S. (1973) *Remedial Drama*. London: Pitman.

Jennings, S. (1999) *Introduction to Developmental Play Therapy*. London: Jessica Kingsley.

Johnson, D.R. (1986) 'The developmental method in drama therapy: Group treatment with the elderly', *The Arts in Psychotherapy*, 33, pp. 17–33.

Johnson, D.R. (2005) *Developmental Transformations: Text for Practitioners*. USA: Author.

Johnson, D.R. (2010) 'Performing Absence: The Limits of Testimony in the Recovery of the Combat Veteran', in Leveton, E. (ed.) *Healing Collective Trauma Using Sociodrama and Drama Therapy*. New York: Springer, pp. 55–80.

Jones, P. (1996) *Drama as Therapy: Theatre as Living.* London & New York: Routledge.

Landy, R. (1982) *Handbook of Educational Drama and Theatre.* Westport: Greenwood.

Lawrence, D.H. (1994) *The Complete Poems of D H Lawrence.* Ware: Wordsworth Editions Ltd.

Lawson, B. (2001) *The Language of Space.* Oxford: Architectural Press.

Mussa, A. (2016) 'I Am a Black Flower: The Use of Rituals in Dramatherapy Work with a Special Education Class in Arab-Israeli Society', in Holmwood, C. and Jennings, S. (eds.) *Routledge International Handbook of Dramatherapy.* London & New York: Routledge, pp. 208–2017.

Parker, R. and Charles, H. (1939) *We'll Meet Again.* London: Michael Ross Ltd.

Pendzik, S. (1994) 'The theatre stage and the sacred space: A comparison', *The Arts in Psychotherapy*, 21(1), pp. 25–35.

Pitruzella, S. (2018) 'The space which divides and connects: Betweenness and the intersubjective perspective', *Dramatherapy*, 39(1), pp. 3–15.

Read, G. (2005) 'Architectural exploration in the théâtre de l'espace (theatre of space) Paris, 1937', *Journal of Architectural Education*, 58(4), pp. 53–62.

Read, G. (2013) 'Introduction: The Play's the Thing', in Feuerstein, M. and Read, G. (eds.) *Architecture As a Performing Art.* Farnham & Burlington: Ashgate, pp. 1–14.

Roose-Evans, J. (1994) *Passages of the Soul.* Rockport: Element Books.

Schrier, C. (2014) 'Young children learn by copying you', *Michigan State University Extension.* Retrieved May 23, 2021, from https://www.canr.msu.edu/news/young_children_learn_by_copying_you

Shakespeare, W. (2007) *Collected Works.* Bate, J. and Rasmussen, E. (eds.). London: Random House.

Slade, P. (1954) *Child Drama.* London: University of London Press.

Turner, V. (1967) *The Forest of Symbols.* New York: Cornell University Press.

Turner, V. (1977). System, and symbol: A new anthropological synthesis, Daedalus, 106, pp. 61–80.

Turner, V. (1982) *From Ritual to Theatre: The Human Seriousness of Play.* New York: PAJ Publications.

Turner, V. (1995) *The Ritual Process: Structure and Anti-Structure.* New York: Aldine de Gruyter.

Van Gennep, A. (1960) *The Rites of Passage.* Chicago: University of Chicago Press.

Winnicott, D. (1994) *Playing and Reality.* New York: Basic Books.

# 11 Preparing the Ritual Space

## The Transition from Everyday Reality to Dramatic Reality

*Drew Bird*

## Introduction

The chapter will consider how setting the scene prepares the psyche for the transition from the everyday experience to a dramatic persona. Using van Gennep's (1960/2004) rite of passages, Joseph Campell's (1988) monomyth and Turner's (2017) ritual process, I will illustrate how they shape and structure a dramatherapy session. I will pay special attention to preparing and transforming the theatre space and therapy space to change the dominant culture of a pre-existing room to create a safe and non-judgemental space. I will explore the importance of ritual threshold crossings that help performer, audience, client and therapist to fully transition from an ordinary to extra-ordinary reality that has the potential to be a sacred space. The word sacred may have religious connotations, however, for Eliade (1959), it was a belief in some kind of 'regenerative power ... that could be tapped into for personal and social regeneration' (Moore, 2001: 27).

Significant in the transition from one reality to another is change and how ritual crossings offer opportunity to experience and process loss and mini deaths (Gersie, 1991) that accompany moving from one space to another. The stage and the therapy space are both sacred spaces that facilitate transformation of the actor, audience, facilitator and client. When an actor enters the stage or a client enters the therapy space, they enter through a doorway, literal or symbolic, that helps to shift their psyche from the profane, secular space, to the sacred (Moore, 2001). There is regenerative and transformational power in the sacred space. Victor Turner (2017) regarded the sacred space as a liminal and temporary space that breaks us free from our everyday lives and roles to undergo true transformation.

## Separating from Everyday Reality

The initiation into the sacred and liminal space starts with separation, the first stage in Van Gennep's (1960/2004) understanding of rites of passage, where separation is leaving behind all that is familiar. I recall when I was ordained as a Buddhist some years ago, leaving the UK and my job for 4 months to live in the Spanish mountains with 20 other men without contact from the outside

DOI: 10.4324/9781003252399-15

world. The separation phase accompanied a sense of dying, that felt very real. I made a will and arrangements for my funeral as there was a strong sense of not knowing whether I would return after four months. On reflection some four years later, I realize there was a sense of spiritual death. I was letting go of familiar roles as a teacher and dramatherapist and entering a sacred and liminal space that was characterized by uncertainty. There was a strong sense that I would not be returning as the person I once was and that I would undergo a significant transformation.

The actor entering the stage also needs to separate from everyday life, engaging in the transition phase (Van Gennep, 1960/2004), rites of passage with a costume and staged set with lights and an audience. In a similar way, the audience also embarks on this process. Entering the theatre requires a separation and threshold crossing into the world of the theatre, where disbelief is suspended and anything can happen.

My fascination for the separation phase in rites of passage was explored in a performance presented at the European Federation of Dramatherapists annual conference in Bucharest in 2016, that explored the links between the personal and professional and how theatre practice informed my development as a dramatherapist. The performance opened with a separation ritual, with the protagonist sweeping the stage space with a broom. The separation ritual was also a preparation ritual that was influenced by Japanese Noh Theatre and Oshi Yoda, which is about cleansing the stage space mindfully (Oida and Marshall, 1997). The ritual was about transforming the everyday classroom space offered for the performance into a sacred space that accompanies a different kind of consciousness. Normally an actor's preparations and warmups take place out of sight of the audience. In my performance, I wanted the cleansing ritual to be part of the performance. I didn't want to separate the preparations out from the performance. Sweeping the space mindfully helped me to concentrate and focus my mind. Sweeping debris from the designated stage space was also about removing the potential of pre-existing charges in the space that normally was used as a classroom. The ritual helped to transform the everyday reality of the room into a stage and sacred space that was suitable for a performance.

## The Conditioned Space

Space imposes its own conditions on the performance, so the ritual was an attempt to break with the conditioned habits of the normal classroom function of the space (Brook, 1987).

I have performed in many different types of spaces. What I have noticed is the impact the space can have on the performance itself. My successful performances took place in more intimate and dark spaces that resembled a cabaret setting. But there have been performances that don't seem to have captured the magic of theatre. I recall one particular performance that took part in a large empty space usually used as a gymnasium. Even though it was packed with an audience, it felt sterile and lacked atmosphere. The conditioned nature of the gymnasium imposed itself on the performance, and as a consequence, I struggled to connect with the audience past the front row. Had we been closer together, I believe our connection and exchange would have been more dynamic. The outcome of the performance had an element of dead theatre about it rather than the holy theatre and magical theatre, where the invisible is made visible (Brook, 1987; Brook, 2008).

In my performance at the University of Bucharest, the audience witnessed my preparations as an actor. In this way, it helped to prepare the audience and free them from the usual conditioned nature of the space and transform it from a classroom to a theatre space. The ritual helped to mark the separation from the familiar, much like van Gennep's (1960/2004) first stage of rites of passage. In this way, the psyche of the space, the audience and the actor were prepared. The cleansing ritual helped to prepare the space into a 'pure, virgin space' that was ready and receptive for some new experience (Brook, 1995: 4). Creating a neutral space that helps the audience to imagine. The simple act of witnessing someone in an empty space is all that is needed for the creation of theatre (Brook, 2008).

Preparing the dramatherapy space needs the same consideration as preparing the theatre space. In my experience as a dramatherapist, I have not offered therapy in a purpose-built space; I have to transform the room's everyday identity into an appropriate, suitable and sacred space for dramatherapy. However, I do feel this has advantages, and transforming and cleansing the space helps with my preparations. Changing the room by moving chairs and tables, removing litter, rolling up the blinds and opening the window to let in the fresh air all help to cleanse the room of its earlier uses and the 'charges' left behind by the earlier occupants.

The room as a potential sacred space in the first instance needs to be respected. In Japanese culture, the act of cleansing and purifying the self and surroundings takes on a spiritual dimension that implies respect and is about preparing oneself in body and mind for the work to be done (Oida and Marshall, 1997). It is important to remember the room is a container for the client's psyche, that art therapist Brown (2008) also considers to be a 'set apart space' and 'sanctuary'. Much like the dramatherapist needs to be fully available to receiving the client, the room also needs to be in an equally receptive state.

Preparing the space for the client helps to prepare the facilitator's psyche, to get them into a therapeutic state of consciousness. By mindfully attending to their body/mind experience, the therapist can become aware of potential psychic contaminations that might impact the therapist's availability for the client. The everyday reality, identity and conditioning of the room will potentially impact the client's feeling safe, contained and free from judgement. As a dramatherapist, I was once offered a head teacher's office for a therapy session in a school, that clearly would not help to cultivate a safe and judgement free space where the client is able to fully express themselves. A classroom, conference room or colleague's office can all have unhelpful conditioning, 'charges', or associations for the client if not suitably transformed. If the client is able to self-actualize, then their basic needs of an appropriate space or 'shelter' need to be met before any other consideration (Maslow, 2014).

Rooms are conditioned with a dominant culture and narrative (White and Epstein, 1990) that are accompanied by 'constructs, beliefs and values' (Bird, 2010: 12) that pose challenges for the therapeutic work. And course, there are some rooms that may not be redeemable for therapy. I recall leading a workshop for practitioners exploring ways to work safely with sexual abuse. The large city hall room was lined with old oil paintings of men with large gold-coloured frames in council costumes staring at us from their positions of power. The pictures were symbolic of the dominant white male gaze and its power structures, and clearly not a safe enough space to develop a trusting and open relationship that was free of judgement. Had I checked out the room in advance, I would never have sanctioned the space. A room of this kind I doubt could be transformed into a suitable therapy space, much like the head teacher's office, so it is important to recognize that not every space can be suitably transformed.

Before the room is fit for purpose, it needs to be neutralized or de-rolled of any charges it might have to make it a suitable space for therapy. The dramatherapy space is a sacred space. I can't help thinking that the therapy is only as good as the room you are in. If the space has not been cared for and tended to, I wonder what this says about the therapist. The space is part of the therapeutic relationship and holding dynamic and forms the tripartite relationship of space, client and therapist, much like the therapist, client and drama dynamic (Jennings, 1999).

## The Liminal Space (Extraordinary Sacred Space)

Whilst initially in the therapeutic work, I prepare the therapeutic space as a facilitator before the client(s) arrives as the work develops, and I like to integrate the preparation of the space into the therapeutic work itself, much like I integrated the cleansing ritual into my performance. The preparation of the space then acts as an opening ritual for the client that intensifies the separation from the everyday experience, acting as a threshold crossing from one reality to another. The threshold crossing is a shift from an everyday, secular or profane to a sacred consciousness. Turner (2017) considered the sacred space to be liminal, where people, or in the case of therapy, the client, relate very differently compared to ordinary ways of being. The client being active in transforming the space helps mark in a concrete way what Campbell (1988) called the call to adventure in the myth of the hero and the desire to transform their life. A safe space according to Rogers (2000: 12) helps the client to 'venture into the land of authenticity' and create a non-judgemental environment for exploration (Levine and Levine, 1999). Empowering the client to transform the space helps them take ownership and develop a more personal relationship with the space. Facilitating the client to imagine the different colours they would like the walls painted, the kind of coverings on the floor and what kind of furniture they would like all help to create a safe space. The transformation ritual helps with the threshold crossing into what Van Gennep (1960/2004) called the transition phase in rites of passage, where the initiate, or in this case, the client in individual work, steps into a new reality where their normal roles and responsibilities are temporarily suspended.

Having the same kind of opening ritual every week makes it easier to see the changes in the client's relationship with the space and the therapeutic process. In a similar way, Yalom (2002) was able to notice changes in his clients as they walked along the same path to his therapy room. Noticing their movement and general demeanour through their body language, he was able to compare and contrast how they walk over time. Having the same space for therapy helps to heighten and see more clearly the changes in the client's relationship with the space, and how the safe and not so safe spaces in the room change week to week. Enabling the client to develop their relationship with the space helps them into a playful relationship with the space, much like Winnicott's (2005) emphasis in psychotherapy is to bring the client into a playful relationship with the therapist.

Facilitating the client into a playful relationship with the space and actively engaging their imagination empowers them to create the kind of conditions they need for change, much like Roger's (1995) belief that given the right conditions, clients can be self-actualizing. Therapy rooms have their own dominant culture that can feel alien and disempowering for a client. When a client creates their own space, they are creating their own unique cultural context and conditions for change and transformation. It is important that the therapist is able to enter into the client's world as represented by the creation of their space. Much like Yalom (2002) considered inventing a new therapy for every client, every client needs to invent their own therapy space. In the same spirit of tailoring a space to client needs, Tipple (2006) argued the art therapy space needs to be adapted to different client groups. Helping clients find and create their idyllic space is akin to Lahad's (1992) approach to six-part story where the therapist aligns with the client's world rather than the client to the therapist's world.

Helping the clients prepare the space helps with the transition from their everyday reality to a different kind of reality. The creation of a safe space helps the client to symbolically master themselves (Winnicott, 2005) when outside the therapy space they may have limited control over their environment. The creation of an imaginary space also symbolically offers clues to the client's needs. A client imagining a space where there is a free vending machine with an inexhaustible supply of crisps and coca cola and bean bags scattered around the room might point to the importance of the client's basic needs being met. Self-actualizing is limited if the basic needs of food, water, warmth, rest, security and safety are not met (Maslow, 2014). It's important to point out here that my approach to dramatherapy and the importance of space as a container is informed by working with children who have experienced abuse and trauma. Neglect, emotional abuse, and fear impact children's basic needs not being met. A space where needs are addressed symbolically and unconsciously can help the client to feel more safe and secure so they can play. Without a sense of safety, play can be inhibited significantly (Gammage, 2017). Facilitating a space of the client's design where they are in control sets up a pre-requisite for playing and experimenting where the fear of reprisals is minimized.

It is important to slow down the processes entering the therapy world as this intensifies the client experience but also allows them processing time as the transition from one space to another. The first threshold is through the therapy door and then preparing the space before the client imagines the kind of space, they want to work in. They are negotiating different thresholds before negotiating the final threshold where they enter the dramatic space. All the thresholds are part of the process of preparation and offer scaffolding for the client so when they do enter the dramatic reality, they are ready to engage.

In a similar way, my performance in Bucharest used the cleansing ritual as a threshold crossing and preparation for the dramatic reality. Once I had completed the cleaning ritual, I then proceed to create the market place scene where the drama was to take place. I had no props or physical scenery, only my imagination and the audiences'. Whilst I proceeded to point out the fruit and vegetable, fresh bread and fish stalls, the outlines offered sufficient structure for the audience to imagine and fill in the details, that encouraged a co-creation (Brook, 2008). My hope was that the audience were more invested because they were potentially active participants in the creation of the scene rather than passive observers. In this way, I was facilitating the audience to take ownership of their creations, aware that everyone in the audience would have created their own unique market scene, stalls and village well. The setting up of the space and scene helps to prepare the psyche for the transition to the imaginary world. Actively facilitating the audience's imagination paradoxically helps to make it more real, especially if you encourage them to detail what they see, much like Stanislavski's (2013) approach to acting. It is the role of the actor, much like that of the facilitator, to facilitate the audience so they can see the chain and the bucket that is hanging over the well. The facilitator and actor are both ritual leaders that help to transform the liminal space and sacred space that tribal and indigenous populations have developed for personal transformation for centuries (Moore, 2001). The roles also resonate with the magician archetype to help 'bring into being what never was there before, about claiming our roles as co-creators of the universe' (Pearson, 1998: x). The Magician's role is to help others see what they can't see (Brook, 2008) and guide the audience and/or clients into a 'ritual initiatory process' (Moore, 2001: 98), guiding the audience through threshold crossings.

In generic dramatherapy practice, I believe there can be a tendency to neglect setting up the scene and moving too quickly to the character development. There is a concern that the setting up of the scene could be relegated and separated from the action of the drama. The setting up of the scene is part of the drama. The scenery and props reinforce the dramatic reality of the scene which reinforces the separateness from the client's everyday reality, but also acts as a container for the characters. The scenic space points to the symbolic conditions and context of the character's life. Everything in the drama is an externalizing of the client's inner world, and this includes the stage set (Jones, 2007), much like everything in the novel, poem or play are all aspects and sub-personalities of the author (Rowan, 1989). The chair, the table and the window are all aspects of the client's psyche pointing to their internal drama. How the client imagines the staged set has the potential to mirror a largescale spectrogram, where the relative positions, colours and shapes symbolically represent the client's inner world.

The threshold crossing from everyday reality to dramatic reality is managed in such a way to heighten the transition and threshold crossing. Enabling the client to imagine what they are crossing helps to intensify their experience and thus help them enter more fully into the dramatic world. The client may imagine a wall of fire, a stream, a sea or even a dessert; the most important thing is that it has meaning for them as they leave one world for another. Stepping into the extraordinary world is what Moore (2001) considers the transition phase (van Gennep, 1960/2004), liminal space (Turner, 2017) and sacred space (Eliade, 2020) to transcend ordinary consciousness where the client's everyday reality is dismantled and deconstructed much like a death that is accompanied by grief. In a psychotherapy context, the space is a vessel or container that helps to create intensity. The conditioning of the new dramatic reality and scene is an opportunity to suspend the client's more usual roles and their accompanying patterns and habits, that can also be disorientating. With all change, there is a sense of loss that is central to the transition phase and transformation process. A clearly imagined scene helps to manage and contain potentially overwhelming experiences as it helps to hold the client much like a mother figure.

Creating a containing scene and environment is akin to good enough parenting that has a predictable element to nurture the child (Winnicott, 2005). The stage manager role in theatre has similarities with the parent role; managing the client's entrance into the dramatic reality. In the theatre, the stage manager manages furniture and props, costumes, supervising the 'get-in' and 'get-out' and calling in the actor so they are prepared to enter the stage at the right time. A predictable structure and ritual for the managing and guiding the client into the drama helps to contain any anxiety so they leave one world for another with the minimal amount of risk. If the client is fully prepared and they have actively imagined the scene, this helps to manage the uncertainty that can accompany visiting a new place as there is a degree of predictability about it. When we visit a new country, we find out as much as we can about it by reading guidebooks so that we can both prepare ourselves for the new and potentially alien experiences in a new culture. In the same way, the client needs to be encouraged to have as much control of creating the dramatic reality by seeing, touching, hearing and smelling what their new world will be like so they can engage more fully and not be overwhelmed with anxiety.

The scene once set is then ready for the character development and the action of the drama will unfold in a form of improvisation that is characterized by uncertainty. In contrast, the scenery is a constant and thus predictable and can act as a secure base that can help manage the uncertainty of the developing drama. The balance between familiarity and uncertainty needs to be carefully managed so the client can take risks, but not to the extent where they may feel overwhelmed. The scene acts as a container to hold the dramatic action in a way so the client can explore the risks that come from an improvised drama. Finding the right balance between containment, familiarity and safety and the risk that accompanies improvisation and uncertainty is important. We are looking for a safe enough space to manage the uncertainty, not remove risk, because risk is important as this helps the client go beyond their current limited understanding and experience.

There may be some situations where the client might not be ready for character development, where the focus of the work is only scene setting. However, there is still dramatic enormous opportunity for exploring the created scene as it is the externalized symbolic inner world of the client. David Grove, counselling psychologist, developed a therapeutic approach that utilized location that he believed held knowledge. The space or location was either inside the body or in perceptual metaphorical space (Dilts and DeLozier, 2000; Lawley and Manea, 2017). The scene is a configuration of the client's inner world that helps the client to access the internalized dynamics and relationships with the different aspects of the self. The world we all live in is the world we have created. There are as many different worlds as their inhabitants in the world we all live in; no two are the same. Similarly, the scene the client has created has the potential to be the world they live in. We configure the outer world, so it mirrors our inner world (Jung, 1964).

The tree, the park bench and the children's roundabout in an imagined scene are all aspects of the self, much like everything in the dream is the dreamer, including inanimate objects (Hillman's dream paper). The externalizing of the client's inner world through a scene offers the client different angles, views and perspectives they might not be able to access so easily if the scene remains internalized. It can be challenging to find a new perspective or spacious relationship with one's inner world as one can become so attached or even stuck with an internalized view. Yet, within an externalized world, a whole array of accessible viewing points becomes possible and easy to navigate (Bird, 2010). The client can view the scene laying down, standing up, hiding behind a tree, sitting on the roundabout, standing on a chair, etc. There are many possibilities. The scene offers a new creative landscape of the client's psyche that can bring the client into a new relationship with their problems (Jones, 2007; Smith and Bird, 2013). When there are different ways of viewing a problem, there is more choice, and consequently, the client can feel more empowered. When the problem is viewed only from one perspective, it can feel oppressive, as choice has been marginalized. Course, we often experience this kind of situation when someone is able to point out another way of looking at a problem that we had not considered before. Offering a client to view the scene in multiple and alternative ways helps to alleviate oppression and expand their repertoire of perspectives (Boal, 1995).

As a therapist, I always proceed with caution and reverence when entering the client's scene as it can be perceived as invasive or abusive. And course, there may be times when it might be inappropriate to inhabit the scene. It is important to recognize that I am a welcome guest into the scene, aware that I am too crossing a threshold from the therapy space into the client's dramatic reality, scene, inner world, sacred space and psychic space. The places in the scene where the client is drawn and places where they might feel aversion represent the places and spaces in the client's psyche, so proceeding with reverence, respect and caution is important.

## Client Vignette

The following case example is not specific to one client, but rather a conglomerate of cases in the form of a fictitious client that captures the themes I have so far explored.

Jez was an 11-year-old boy who presented at his primary school as timid and anxious. He had one close friend but struggled in a social group. In six months' time, he was due to move from a primary school to a senior secondary school.

The only spare room in the school was a classroom in Jez's school. It was not his usual classroom, but Jez did have a previous relationship with the classroom.

On entering the room, Jez had sat in a chair behind the children's tables. I wondered whether there was an expectation from Jez that I sat behind the teacher's desk. It felt important right from the start to make clear that I am not a teacher, but a therapist, so I pulled up one of the children's chairs and sat beside him, causing him to smile. Sometimes nonverbal communication of this kind can have more impact than words.

I told Jez we were going to change the classroom into a therapy room. I started to move the tables and chairs to create the space as Jez watched on. Jez responded with a little trepidation at my invitation to help me, but nonetheless, he started to help. We created a space of about 7 m². I suggested we cover the tables with fabrics from the bag, inviting Jez to choose the fabrics that he liked the colour, touch and smell of before together creating a more personalized ritual space that was certainly different from the usual classroom space. The therapy space looked more contained, compared to the large classroom. Sat on cushions Jez and I were less visible to the large window. I noticed there was something different in Jez's demeanour, perhaps more relaxed, or curious, whatever it was, there was a change in his physical pre-sentation. Jez commented that the space felt like a den. I helped him elaborate further, where he established it was a secret den. I also noticed a change in myself, I felt more at ease too in the new environment, aware of the impact the classroom may have had on activating my conditioning with early school and my then identity as a troublesome boy.

It felt like the therapy space started to activate Jez's imagination, so together we co-created a story about a main character called Tick who built a den in the forest to hide. Jez described the forest as dark with large trees and together we developed the sound of the forest. I was aware that the forest could have many symbolic meanings, one of these could have been his up-coming new school. I suggested to Jez that he could bring anything he could imagine into the therapy space. Jez developed a bag that produced an inexhaustible supply of sweets and chocolate, aware that these had the potential to provide Jez with symbolic resources to help him face any potential fears outside of the therapy space we had created. Jez's suggestion also helped me to ascertain that he had created a space that was free from the school rule conditioning. I reinforce that the therapy space was not a classroom so we could eat as many sweets and chocolates as we liked. Playfully we gorged on the delights.

My hope was that the sweets and chocolates helped to reinforce the play-fulness of the therapy space, but it was also important that the space was thoroughly deroled and the rules of the classroom returned at the end of the therapy session, so that Jez was not confused post-therapy.

After a rather lengthy improvisation and play around the different sweets and chocolates we were eating that went from everyday sweets to our own mirac-ulous inventions with magical properties, I started to close the session down. Initially, Jez seemed reluctant to leave the den behind. After a while, he said, 'Do we have to? I like it here'. It was important that there was plenty of time to permit a slow and considered return from the therapy space to Jez's everyday world and the classroom. Jez needed time to process his return safely. Initially, Jez sat whilst I started to pile up the cushions and take the fabrics down. I was in no rush to yank Jez from the therapy space and drop him unprepared into the classroom. There was plenty of time, so I was able to fold up the fabrics and put them into the bag one at a time. I deliberately took my time because, as Jez witnessed this, I surmised that he was potentially processing the end of the session. After doing this several times, I picked a larger fabric and asked Jez if he wanted to help me fold it, to which he appeared receptive. As we folded up the fabrics, I proceeded to thank the den for helping us to imagine and again help Jez with the transition, aware it could have had symbolic representations of the primary school he would be leaving soon.

We continued dismantling and deroling the space by moving the chairs and tables back to their usual places. I checked in with Jez how the classroom looked. All he was able to say was that it seemed different but didn't elaborate further on this. Everything in the room had returned to its usual state, but something had changed for Jez. I imagined his relationship with the class-room was different in some way. Before fully leaving the space, we talked about the maths class Jez was returning to. He didn't like maths, but the more we talked about maths, the more prepared I felt he was for a return to the classroom next door. At the end of conversation about maths, we proceeded to leave the classroom and make our goodbyes until the next session.

As illustrated in this case example, this work enabled Jez to explore his relationship with the large classroom/dark forest and master his play with the different spaces and all their potential symbolism and confusion. However, despite the potential symbolic possibilities, these were only made possible by having clear concrete boundaries in the physical setting up of the therapy space and delineating it as separate from the classroom space.

The deroling also had the potential to help Jez prepare to leave his current school in a symbolic and indirect way. The co-creative process of setting up a new space and deroling the space also offered Jez support. He was not left on his own, I was alongside him, making the changes with him. The co-creation also helped me transition myself fully from the classroom to the therapy space so I could be fully present to support him.

Returning Jez safely to the maths class was essential so he could fully inhabit being in the role of a school pupil again, with all its challenges for him. A successful return to maths was as important, so Jez's imagination was kept appropriately contained and not spilling out in the maths lesson.

## Preparing for the Return to Everyday Reality

Leaving the scene behind is also a threshold crossing and marks the beginning of reintegration. The journey back from the dramatic reality to the client's everyday reality marks the 'return' in Campbell's (1988) monomyth, incorporation in van Gennep's (1960/2004) rites of passage and Turner's (2017) post-liminal stage. Within a psychotherapy frame, this reconstituting of ordinary consciousness and reintegration is the post-analysis adaption (Moore, 2001). I am aware that I support and enable the client to return from an altered state of consciousness to everyday consciousness, aware of the potential for disorientation, where the client is sensitive, receptive and needs support. Turner (2017) warns of a 'liminoid' phase where there has been a false initiation, as in soldiers, where there is a failure to psychologically bring them home. The 'liminoid' space is not contained by a ritual, and consequently, transformation is limited. Whilst the liminal space is different where ritual leaders hold and contain the space so that transformation can occur (Moore, 2001). In the same manner in dramatherapy, the client needs to have been initiated into the dramatic space, so they can have a carefully managed return from the space from the facilitator. As the threshold crossing into the dramatic space enrols the client into the scene, the return threshold crossing marks a deroling. According to Landy (1992), derolment is a death, where the client navigates the change from the potential within the dramatic reality, returning to an everyday reality with its self-limiting beliefs and limitations. The systematic deroling of the tree, bench and roundabout in the scene is important even if they are imagined. It is important that the scene is closed down as this offers the opportunity to have a closure and enables the client to have an experience of loss. Yalom (2002) encourages therapists to explore death with their clients as death anxiety can play a role in a client's pathology. Intensifying the return threshold crossing helps the clients to process the change, loss and death so they can become more accustomed and robust with the many mini deaths throughout daily living (Gersie, 1991) and embrace the fullness of the lived experience of being human.

Whilst deroling the dramatic scene is important, the created therapy space also needs to be deroled. Returning the imagined coloured walls, carpet and furniture, and any other physical changes to the room, is also important as it helps to close and contain the therapeutic work, like putting on a symbolic lid onto a pan. The closing ritual helps with the adaption from therapeutic work to everyday that helps the client process this experience. Like all threshold crossings, it is important they are not rushed, aware of the client's return and incorporation into the community they left earlier to embark on a session of therapy. It is important as I stressed earlier with Turners (2017) liminoid phase that the client is returned safely and able to adjust to the demands of a life that awaits them beyond the therapy space. The return to ordinary everyday consciousness is a challenge, but careful stage management can help the client integrate their discoveries into their everyday life. Moore (2001: 186) considers how a successful return phase after a session of therapy can be accompanied by 'enhanced personal status' and 'powers of personal agency reaffirmed'. This might appear a somewhat idealist expectation for therapy after every session, but over the course of therapy, the client needs to be feel more empowered and have more agency and autonomy.

## Conclusion

Leaving and entering the different kinds of spaces that the client embarks on throughout dramatherapy helps them master the new consciousness that accompanies the different spaces. A careful and considered return as a rite of passage can be contrary to one's usual experience, where often the significant events of one's life are overlooked as the pace of life seems to get faster and faster and the processing of experience can be easily overlooked. It is important that the set aside and sacred space of therapy does not mirror the urgency that the information age and its accompanying technology seem to generate. It is important as therapists that we can stage manage the client's transition from one space to another so they can process their experience in a meaningful way, aware of how each threshold crossing has the potential to carry many symbolic meanings that can be missed. If we do not permit the client time to process their experience as therapists, we are in danger of facilitating another liminoid experience for the client.

## References

Bird, D. (2010) 'The power of a new story: The bigger picture. Narrative therapy and the role of aesthetic distance within the process of re-authoring in dramatherapy', *Dramatherapy*, 31(3), pp. 10–14.

Boal, A. (1995) *The Rainbow of Desire: The Boal Method of Theatre and Therapy*. London: Routledge.

Brown, C. (2008) 'Very toxic. Handle with care. Some aspects of maternal function in art therapy', *Inscape*, 13(1), pp. 13–24.

Brook, P. (1987) *The Shifting Point: 40 Years of Theatrical Exploration 1946–1987*. London: Methuen Drama.

Brook, P. (1995) *There Are No Secrets: Thoughts on Acting and Theatre*. London: Bloomsbury.

Brook, P. (2008) *The Empty Space*. London: Penguin Classics.

Campbell, J. (1988) *The Hero with a Thousand Faces*. London: Paladin.

Dilts, R. and DeLozier, J. (2000) *Encyclopedia of Systemic NLP and NLP New Coding*. Santa Cruz, CA: NLP University Press.

Eliade, M. (1959) *The Sacred and the Profane: The Nature of Religion*. London: Elsevier Health.

Eliade, M. (2020) *Shamanism: Archaic Techniques of Ecstasy*. First Princeton Classics Paperwork Printing.

Gammage, D. (2017) *Playful Awakening: Releasing the Gift of Play in Your Life*. London: JKP.

Gersie, A. (1991) *Storymaking in Bereavement: Dragons Flight in the Meadow*. London: Jessica Kingsley.

Jennings, S. (1999) *Introduction to Developmental Playtherapy: Playing and Health*. London: Jessica Kingsley.

Jones, P. (2007) *Drama as Therapy Volume 1: Theory, Practice and Research*. 2nd ed. Hove, East Sussex: Routledge.

Jung, C. (1964) *Man and His Symbols*. London: Picador.

Lahad, M. (1992) 'Storymaking in Assessment Method for Coping with Stress', in Jennings, S. (ed.), *Dramatherapy Theory and Practice 2*. London: Routledge, pp. 150–163.

Landy, R. (1992) 'The drama therapy role method', *Dramatherapy*, 14(2), pp. 7–15.

Lawley, J. and Manea, A.I. (2017) 'The use of clean space to facilitate a "stuck" client- A case study', *Journal of Experiential Psychotherapy*, 20(4), p. 80.

Levine, S.K. and Levine, E.G. (1999) *Foundations of Expressive Arts Therapy*. London: Jessica Kingsley.

Maslow, A. (2014) *A Theory of Human Motivation*. Floyd, VA: Sublime Books.

Moore, R.L. (2001) *The Archetype of Initiation: Sacred Space, Ritual Process, and Personal Transformation. Lectures and Essays by Robert L. Moore*. USA: Xlibris.

Oida, Y. and Marshall, L. (1997) *The Invisible Actor*. London: Methuen.

Pearson, C. (1998) *The Hero Within: Six Archetypes We Live By*. New York, NY: HarperSanFrancisco.

Rogers, C.R. (1995) *A Way of Being: The Founder of the Human Potential Movement Looks Back on a Distinguished Career*. New York, NY: Houghton Mifflin Company.

Rogers, N. (2000) *The Creative Connection: Expressive Arts as Healing*. Monmouth, IL: PCCS Books.

Rowan, J. (1989) *Subpersonalities: The People Inside Us*. London: Routledge.

Smith, M.E., and Bird, D. (2013). 'Fairy tales, landscapes and metaphor in supervision: An exploratory study'. *Counselling and Psychotherapy Research.* 10.1080/14733145.2013.779732

Stanislavski, C. (2013) *Building a Character.* London: Bloomsbury.

Tipple, R. (2006) 'The Art Therapy Room', in Case, C. and Dalley, T. (eds.), *Handbook of Art Therapy.* 2nd ed. London: Routledge.

Turner, V. (2017) *The Ritual Process: Structure and Anti-Structure.* London: Routledge.

Van Gennep, A. (1960/2004) *The Rites of Passage.* London: Routledge.

White, M. and Epstein, D. (1990) *Narrative Means to Therapeutic End.* New York, NY: Norton and Company.

Winnicott, D.W. (2005) *Playing and Reality.* Great Britain: Routledge Classic Edition.

Yalom, I. (2002) *The Gift of Therapy: Reflections on Being a Therapist.* London: Piatkus Books.

# Postlude

## Future Spaces of Dramatherapy

*Eliza Sweeney*

It is fitting that as we opened this volume with a prelude, we should close with a postlude, commonly understood to be a short musical piece that concludes a performance. Written text is a wonderfully rich medium and in an academic sense, it is very useful in documenting one's thoughts and a critical examination of a subject in a commonly understood language (in this case written English and using dramatherapy vocabulary). However, as with all expressive and artistic mediums, we understand the limits of the written language. It prevents those who do not speak the common shared language employed in a text from directly accessing the information and it restricts embodied expressions of play, song, dance, theatrical interpretation or musical interludes. Had I been able, I should have liked to improvise a rhythmic chant in celebration of this concluding moment together. A dramatic ritual to close. In my search for a happy compromise, I invite you to play some music while you venture through this concluding piece, at the end of the volume of a text written by such a rich variety of professional voices across the globe. Even though we have arrived at the end, I venture to suggest that while a postlude assumes a denouement, a closure, I propose that this postlude be accepted not as a finitude but as a pause in time allowing for quiet reflection. Moreover, I invite you to read it as an opening to new future spaces in dramatherapy, new landscapes and fresh horizons. Following on from the nourishing work that was proposed in the preceding chapters, it is with such an intention that I propose to use this postlude space to discuss two less visited terrains of dramatherapy: the online space and, the most urgent, the ecological crisis.

Before we go forward, however, let us look back and pause to reflect. This book was born of a deep appreciation for the impact of space and place on human lives and grew out of a collective desire to voice thoughts, feelings, experiences and ideas about space in dramatherapy, a subject too lightly touched upon. As scenographer scholar, Arnold Aronson has stated *we are spatial creatures* (Aronson, 2005, p. 1) and the work in this volume is enshrouded by the belief that '*where* things happen is critical to knowing *how* and *why* they happen' (Warf and Arias, 2014). As dramatherapists, we are spatial beings, making, shaping and transforming imaginary, liminal, emotional, relational and psychological spaces as we go. This volume hoped to

DOI: 10.4324/9781003252399-16

illuminate the importance of space and place in our discipline and in doing so, the chapters have ventured to discuss a variety of options to cover an expanse of possibilities: scenographic and architectural space, mask space, hut space, play space, educational space, neuropsychological space, ritual and spiritual space and many more. In this world of divides, closures, confinements and restrictions of physical closeness, we have attempted (and I venture to suggest successfully achieved) to provide a communal space to reunite, to build bridges, cross borders, fill gaps and unite in one place. Reflecting back, I acknowledge just how great a challenge editing this book was. When I began, I wasn't quite sure what would come out of it, or how mountainous the work would be. Ignorance was indeed bliss in this instance as I personally navigated parenting responsibilities of young children, the pandemic and the beginnings of my PhD while editing this volume. While it was a challenge, most of all it was a great privilege. It was a privilege to have carried forth the sacred places and stories of all these contributors and their clients, a privilege to shape them into a coherent structure that provides a space for *spatial* reflection in our discipline. Of course, I acknowledge the limits of one volume and that while we were able to cover many spaces in dramatherapy in this text, a single volume alone could not do justice to such a complex terrain for discussion. Thus, some subject matter was unable to be traversed in this book, for ex-ample online and digital spaces of dramatherapy and the spaces of the eco-logical crisis, which I now propose to consider in some further detail.

Art therapy's early encounter with the digital came in various forums and spaces, by being discussed as a discipline on the internet before becoming a digital clinical practice. The internet has been drawing new frontiers (and closing down other ones) for clinical psychology, art therapy and, more recently, dramatherapy, as the pandemic demonstrated. Dramatherapist Ditty Dokter remarked in the introduction that an insufficient amount has been discussed on digital spaces and dramatherapy highlighting her desire to see more. Volume 6 of The Drama Therapy Review published a special issue of a series of articles on digital dramatherapy interventions in response to growing and unprecedented moves to online platforms to conduct educational, healthcare and therapeutic interventions with submissions covering concerns, personal experience and challenges relating to digital dramatherapy and tel-ehealth interventions (Atsmon and Pendzik, 2020; Sajnani, 2020; Stavrou, 2020; Wood *et al.*, 2020; Rothman, Offerman and Trottier, 2022). The number of respected colleagues who contributed to that volume demonstrates to me that this is a seriously considered space in the dramatherapy realm that has warranted discussion and perhaps warrants further investigation. My own venture into the digital world of dramatherapy occurred during the Covid pandemic and a part of this was documented in the book, *Interiors in the Era of Covid: Interior Design between the Public and Private Realms* (Scholze *et al.*, 2022). Written in collaboration with architect and scholar Sebastian Messer, this chapter discusses how design practices were coupled with narrative concepts and provided a way for clients to *voyage* beyond the confines of the home-space during the pandemic. Drawing upon my work as a dramatherapist and knowledge of role play, storytelling, imagination and my specific technique through which my clients create hut-spaces as therapeutic and creative mediums, I was able to 'reconceive the domestic interior, supporting the mental health and wellbeing of children in precarious socioeconomic circumstances' (Scholze *et al.*, 2022). While this volume was unable to include in-depth reflections upon one or the many digital spaces within the dramatherapy discipline, it is worthy of note here in the postlude as a reminder that as we venture forward towards new horizons in dramatherapy, we continue to reflect upon and critique *other* spaces of dramatherapy, tangible and virtual, that propel us forward into new and possible futures.

In the introduction, I suggested that this volume's intention is to encourage dramatherapists to go *beyond* current ways of practicing, thinking and theorizing dramatherapy into new spaces and places of practice. Online spaces constitute one such new space of practice that many dramatherapy professionals were confronted with during the global coronavirus pandemic. With the pandemic came about new conclusions about the way in which we inhabit our world, our private and our public spheres of life. The pandemic also illuminated the increasing risk to human and non-human life as a direct result of the global ecological crisis (destruction of habitats leads to the closing in of spaces between humans and animals, the collapse of biodiversity results in a reduction of species and therefore increased risk of human contamination and the effect of globalization resulted in the rapid diffusion of the virus, etc.). Going beyond the pages and into the future is a calling for a continual rethinking and re-feeling of space and place for the world of tomorrow. In reference to design practices, scholar Rachel Hann has suggested within the seminal publication *Ecoscenography* by Tanja Beer that 'to design for the feelings that have no name is to design for a period of human civilization that has no precursor' (Beer, 2021). In the current global ecological crisis that we find ourselves in today, I propose that it is time for dramatherapy as a discipline to re-design for this new civilization, to grow from its rich and powerful history where such good work has been accomplished – some of which is presented in this book – and to now go *beyond* current practices. I propose that we begin strong and deep conversations about how we practice differently in this changing world with a specific focus on ecology, on how dramatherapy not only seeks to transform and heal human worlds but the more-than-human as well, to seed thoughts and future practices of dramatherapy that respond to these *feeling that have no name* within the global ecological crisis.

Various scientific literature and research conclude on the importance of taking into account the effects of the ecological crisis on mental health (Clayton *et al.*, 2017; Panu, 2020), but it is difficult for mental health workers including dramatherapists, to mobilize on these subjects without having been made aware of them themselves (Sinanian, 2023). In fact, faced with the ecological emergency, the question as to whether we are *up to solving the problem* (ibid.) is posed. In such a small space this postlude is definitely not up to the task of elucidating with sufficient depth and detail, the details of the increasing urgency of the ecological crisis for our discipline to which we as urgently need to respond. Nevertheless, in the wake of all the work that has been created over the years by the international dramatherapy community, I wish to encourage new spaces of dialogue in our discipline that take us *beyond* current discourses and practices and that respond to *spatial*, environmental (both internal and external) and ecological threats to the human and more-than-human worlds. The global environmental crisis does not threaten us on an individual and direct level for most of the Global North (we are not affected *as sensorially* by the ecological crisis as say, citizens of Pakistan, awash with devastating floods) but primarily it affects us by assaulting the frameworks on which we have built our world or our idea of the world (political, laws, social systems, economic systems, etc.), often accessed via the media. As these external frameworks begin to crumble in synchronicity with ecological erosion, we can see a weathering of internal landscapes accompanying this catastrophe, corrosions which must be responded to in a clinical way, a response that I strongly suggest dramatherapists can provide.

At the time of writing this volume, my current doctoral research in architecture – framed by the ecological crisis – is seeking art and drama therapeutic responses to such questions with a focus on therapeutic design processes. It seeks to investigate the therapeutic potential of design processes in response to individual or collective *feelings of world* that foster transformative emotional, psychological or social outcomes through a process of designing, making and experiencing *affective environments*. As a doctoral researcher and within my relatively privileged position as a dramatherapist in France – where the ecological crisis affects me at a distance (I read shocking accounts on my iPhone from the comfort of my living room which is nothing compared to the reality of a local Australian who has had their home burned to the ground in recent bush fire disasters, for example), I have albeit become increasingly conscious of and feel the emotional, social, political and psychological impact of the ecological crisis and how it affects and effects myself, my client groups and my practice methods. In observing the current trends of spatial and *placial* thinking across interdisciplinary fields for the past 10 years (architecture, geography, anthropology, psychology, etc.), I have noticed a shift in many disciplines towards re-examining what they mean by the definitions they attribute to their disciplines and re-examining of practice, in the face of the ecological crisis. Taking the expanded remit of scenography as an example (for this is one that I know relatively well), we will be able to see parallels with dramatherapy. Scenography began as a theatre-centric discipline concerned entirely with set design, scenic painting and lighting. Similarly, dramatherapy began with what I suggest are 'actor-centric' tools such as improvisation and role play. Both are derived from the theatre and dramaturgical systems. Yet what we are seeing today is not a scenography that belongs only to the theatre, but a scenography that belongs to and participates in the world, with the steady acceptance that scenography exists everywhere and can be anything.

Current practices of expanded scenography demonstrate this broader thinking situated within the ecological crisis as exemplified in Tanja Beer's contribution to eco-scenography (Beer, 2021) for example, where the *processes of making* are pulled into question and the design intentions are ecologically focussed. In wider fields that intersect design and social justice questions, international conferences in architecture, performance design, cultural geography and scenography (to name a few) are in a constant state of shifting and re-defining what they mean by their practices and how they situate themselves in the context of global emergencies and, moreover, they seek to push the contemporary questions of the ecological crisis in challenging and innovative ways. The Saint Etienne Design Biennale (2022) in France is one example, this year's subject focus being on *bifurcation* as it looked towards design innovation in diverting ways, that are future focussed and that consider climate and other global crises. And while we see such *bifurcation* occurring across a myriad of disciplines, where taking the ecological crisis into account has become almost mandatory, I find myself feeling disappointed and deeply frustrated when I read of current or up-and-coming conferences and publications in our dramatherapy community that appear to have yet to grasp the urgency of the climate crisis and our need to respond, seemingly skirting around the subject or revisiting *over-cooked* topics such as role, imagination, creativity, play space, etc. I am bewildered and concerned that in the face of global pandemics and climate emergencies, the ways in which we work as dramatherapy clinicians and artists in this *new world* of the Anthropocene is not (seemingly) the top priority on a list of topics for conversation. Drama therapy is a beautiful, deep and resource-full practice and drama therapists from all cultures have rich and useful skills that can be drawn upon in response to the ecological crisis and that can be built upon to propose new frames and methodologies of working or tools to respond to the mountain of feeling surrounding this subject matter. I have thus taken this privileged opportunity given to me to write a postlude for this book and I am using it as a space to call to adventure all drama therapists, to look to the future. I am using this moment in space and time to reflect and feel about the ecological crisis in relation to the dramatherapy discipline and to raise the alarm for everyone to go beyond what we currently understand in theory and practice and open a space for discussion on this critical topic in our discipline.

What is clear from discussions with colleagues in varying fields across psychology, dramatherapy, creative art therapies and expressive arts therapies, is that no one has all the answers on how to respond to an ecological crisis. It is a collective crisis and therefore, as with many collective crises, it is difficult to hold distance with the issue, as we would perhaps another type of pathology or crisis with which we are not directly associated. In a recent publication on ecopoeisis and expressive arts therapies (Levine and Kopytin, 2022), I stated that the climate crisis calls for creative approaches to understand the influence of the arts on mental health and to better comprehend humanity's apparent detachment from its place in ecological systems. Creative approaches that do not exclude but have yet to sufficiently include dramatherapy. I certainly do not have all the answers, but I do believe that a first and essential step forward is that we need to start looking beyond the past in dramatherapy practices and begin creating new ones that respond to this new world with specific focus on ecology in crisis, a world in peril.

It was my intention that this volume be the opening of a new space to look at dramatherapy practice in a new light, with a focus on how the spaces and places around us can lead to transformation. And I conclude with the suggestions that from here, perhaps we can consider how we might create dramatherapy spaces that respond to the ecological crisis, that respond to the urgent call for healing in an environment that is slowly eroding before our eyes. As Martin Heiddeger suggested, the way in which we inhabit the world and relate to the environment can be viewed as an extension of our identity. In this way, I suggest that dramatherapists can call to question how we identify and how we inhabit, as both citizens of the world but also in our capacity and our privileged positions as therapists, this new world through our practice. Thus, I suggest that dramatherapists who are trained and capable of providing safe, healing, therapeutic spaces, do so in response to increasingly difficult world phenomena. Dramatherapists who in their daily practice provide safe havens, containing and holding spaces and engage with artistic tools to imagine and create new and possible worlds, are most well equipped to provide creative spaces within which we may begin to address some of these anguishes.

In conclusion, I wonder: what place can the dramatherapist take alongside other scientific fields in responding to the ecological crisis and social, individual, political, and collective *pathologies* that may or may not arise? In the era of the Anthropocene dramatherapists will have to be more at the bedside of societies (Sinanian, 2023) to think about the effects and origins of the ecological crisis, not only from the angle of individual or social suffering but as revealing of human-nature dichotomies (Laidlaw and Beer, 2018, p. 283), which is becoming *pathological*. Dramatherapists have a responsibility to consider how we work in response to the ecological crisis and to put in place interventions that are playful and ethically sound.

To conclude in a *preludial* manner, the words of poet Mary Oliver remind us that we are on the threshold of new potentials in our field, these words remind us to attune ourselves to these potentials: *just pay attention, then patch a few words together ... .. this [is] the doorway into ... a silence in which another voice may speak* (Oliver, 2006).

I hope that responses and voices to the ecological crisis will become more pronounced from within our discipline, as creative responses and deep attention to this global emergency are called for. The voices in this volume represent only a small pool of the many varied voices that could be and should be heard on the subject of space and place in dramatherapy and as this book closes, as it must, I continue to hope that new voices will join the conversation and we will continue to build and share in collective shared-space for time to come.

## Bibliography

Aronson, A. (2005) *Looking Into the Abyss: Essays on Scenography*. Ann Arbor: University of Michigan Press (Theater--theory/text/performance).

Atsmon, A. and Pendzik, S. (2020) 'The clinical use of digital resources in drama therapy: An exploratory study of well-established Practitioners', *Drama Therapy Review*, 6(1), pp. 7–26. Available at: 10.1386/dtr_00013_1

Beer, T. (2021) *Ecoscenography: An Introduction to Ecological Design for Performance*. Cham: Palgrave Macmillan.

Clayton, S. *et al.* (2017) *Mental Health and our Changing Climate: Impacts, implications, and guidance*. American Psychological Association, Climate for Health and EcoAmerica.

Laidlaw, B. and Beer, T. (2018) 'Dancing to (re)connect: Somatic dance experiences as a medium of connection with the more-than-human', *Choreographic Practices*, 9(2), pp. 283–309. Available at: 10.1386/chor.9.2.283_1

Levine, S.K. and Kopytin, A.I. (eds.) (2022) *Ecopoiesis: A New Perspective for the Expressive and Creative Arts Therapies in the 21st Century*. London: Jessica Kingsley Publishers.

Oliver, M. (2006) *Thirst: Poems*. 1st ed. Boston: Beacon Press.

Panu, P. (2020) 'Anxiety and the ecological crisis: An analysis of eco-anxiety and climate anxiety', *Sustainability*, 12(19), p. 7836. Available at: 10.3390/su12197836

Rothman, A., Offerman, E. and Trottier, D.G. (2022) 'H.E.R.O. unmasking: A mixed methods pilot study to explore the impact of a tele-drama therapy protocol on frontline healthcare workers during COVID-19', *Drama Therapy Review*, 8(2), pp. 213–233. Available at: 10.1386/dtr_00107_1

Sajnani, N. (2020) 'Digital interventions in drama therapy offer a virtual playspace but also raise concern', *Drama Therapy Review*, 6(1), pp. 3–6. Available at: 10.1386/dtr_00012_2.

Sinanian, A. (2023). "La crise écologique comme miroir de nous-même. Des discours autour de l'éco-anxiété aux angoisses, dénis et pulsions destructrices". Journal de Psychologues. Paris. URL de cet article. https://www.jdpsychologues.fr/article/la-crise-ecologique-comme-miroir-de-nous-meme-des-discours-autour-de-l-eco-anxiete-aux

Scholze, J. *et al.* (eds.) (2022) *Interiors in the Era of COVID: Interior Design between the Public and Private Realms*. 1st edition. London [England]: Bloomsbury Visual Arts.

Stavrou, D. (2020) 'The medium is the message: The transformation of drama therapy practice during COVID-19', *Drama Therapy Review*, 6(2), pp. 97–101. Available at: 10.1386/dtr_00051_1

Warf, B. and Arias, S. (eds.) (2014) *The Spatial Turn: Interdisciplinary Perspectives*. 1. Issued in Paperback. London: Routledge (Routledge studies in human geography, 26).

Wood, L.L. *et al.* (2020) 'Challenges and strategies delivering group drama therapy via telemental health: Action research using inductive thematic analysis', *Drama Therapy Review*, 6(2), pp. 149–165. Available at: 10.1386/dtr_00025_1

# Index

Aesculapian temple 153
agency 2, 21, 36, 48, 50, 57, 62, 92, 108,
    112, 173; voice and 104, 106,
    109–110
*Akasha* 124, 127–129, 134–135
Alaimo, Stacey 50
Alexander, Eben 127; *Proof of Heaven* 126
Alfassa, Mirra 86
Anzieu, Didier 54, 56
Apergi, Atalandi 154
Arias, S. 10
Aristotle 5, 17
Aroha 39, 40n10
Artaud, Antonin 154
Asclepius 153
Attigui, Patricia 51
Aurobindo, Sri 86
autonomy 19, 22–23, 25, 93, 173
Ayurveda 123, 127

Bachelard, Gaston 18, 20, 22, 25–27,
    150; *The Poetics of Space* 19, 149
Baim, C. 69–70
Baima, Timothy 65
Barker, Roger 44
Beer, Tanja 178; *Ecoscenography* 178
behaviour 3–4, 7–8, 31, 44–47, 49, 55,
    58, 80, 82, 107–108, 110, 113,
    144; aggressive 53–54; feelings
    and 99; human 91, 94; self-
    injurious 81; violent 53
Berry, P. 21–22, 26; *Echo's subtle body:
    Contribution to an archetypal
    psychology* 21
Bhabha, Homi 10
*bifurcation* 180
Birot, Pierre Albert 11
Blake, William 20, 126, 140
Bosnak, Robert 60, 62

*Brahman* 129
bridging space 112–113; *see also* space
Brown, C. 164
Buber, Martin 143
Buddhist 123, 127–129, 131, 162
Butler, Jason 84–86

Campbell, J. 165, 172
Case, C. 30
Cattanach, A. 31, 33, 35, 38
Cavarero, Adriana 22
Celenza, A. 2
Chesner, Anna 9–10, 151
Chown, Mary 78
Churchill, Winston 8
Clarke, Isabel 126
Clavel 5
communication 22, 47–48, 64; nonverbal
    170; physical 61; postural 61
community 33, 38, 46, 56, 62, 78, 104,
    152–154, 173, 180; international
    dramatherapy 179; therapeutic 9, 63
consciousness 43, 127–128, 135, 163;
    dual 66; natural 151; ordinary
    168, 172–173; potential state of
    67; sacred 165; therapeutic state
    of 164; threshold 126, 149
consistency 97, 107–108, 110
Cook, Caldwell 83
Cook, E. 45
Covid-19 pandemic 29–30, 34, 36, 40,
    88, 135, 152, 177
Crouch, David 1

Dalley, T. 30
De Angulo, Jaime, *Indian Tales* 137
de Balzac, Honoré, *The unknown
    masterpiece (Le Chef-d'oeuvre
    Inconnu)* 21

defence mechanisms 92
Dening, Greg, *Performances* 124
Descartes, René 5, 145
*Deus sive Natura* 145
developmental appropriateness 98
developmental transformations (DvT)
    157–159
Doel, Marcus 42
Dokter, D. 76–78, 177
Domash, L. 68
Down's Syndrome 82
drama 18–19, 22, 37, 75–77, 79, 83,
    115–116, 137–138, 143, 147,
    149, 151–155, 167–169;
    educational 78, 84–85, 87–88;
    psychological 87; therapy 6, 8,
    10, 180
dramatherapy 40, 91; client spaces in 80;
    concept of space in practice of
    150–151; environments 42;
    group 30, 37, 39, 44, 63–64,
    112–113, 158; intersubjective
    side of 141–142; play in 76–77;
    practice 23, 25, 57, 60, 86, 108,
    115, 123–126, 130, 135, 181;
    realm 177; sessions 30, 36, 43,
    49, 54, 60–61, 65–67, 69, 76, 97,
    114, 130, 149, 157, 162; setting
    57, 62, 70; space and education
    83–86; space and ritual in
    151–153; spiritual side of
    142–144; work 46–47, 49, 67
*Dramatherapy and the New Paradigm*,
    2013 126

Echo 17–22, 27; workshop 18, 23–26
ecological crisis 176–181; global 178
Ekman, Paul 61
Elam, K. 75
El Wardany, H. 153
Embodied Dreamwork 60, 63, 66
Embodied Imagination theory 62–63
embodiment 19, 60, 63, 66, 68, 76–77,
    135, 152; symbolic 77
Embodiment-Projection-Role (EPR)
    model 19, 32, 77
empathy 68–69, 94, 97, 102, 142; and
    distancing 85
Erickson, E. 98
Erskine, R. 97

Fenichel, Otto 3
Fenner, Patricia 8–10, 55–57

Ferrer, J. N. 86
First World War 21
Fordham, Michael 3, 43
Freud, Sigmund 2–4, 10, 62, 92

Gaines, Andrew 84
Gaines, Eliot, *Communication and the
    Semantics of space* 6
Gammage, D. 92, 99
God/Nature 145
Goethe, Johann Wolfgang von 126
Grainger, Roger 25, 39–40, 45,
    137–138, 147, 150–153; *Ritual
    and Theatre* 125
Graziano, Michael S. A. 144
'Ground of Being' 127
Grove, David 169

Hall, Edward T. 6, 8
Hann, Rachel 3, 178; 'Beyond
    Scenography' 10
Hart, Roy 21
Heathcote, Edwin 7
Heidegger, M. 5–6; *The Origin of the
    Work of Art* 130
Holmwood, C. 153
*Hsu* 129
humanity 6, 151, 180
Hurssel, Edmund 5

IDBP *see* Integral Drama Based Pedagogy
identity 21, 25, 38, 153–154, 164, 171,
    181; group 6, 33, 47–48, 56–57;
    personal 142; professional 43;
    therapist 6
imaginal space 113–115; *see also* space
imaginative life 51
imaginative space 112; *see also* space
inmates 64–70, 139, 141; male 63
Integral Drama Based Pedagogy
    (IDBP) 86
intersubjectivity 19, 25, 141, 149–150
*I-Thou* 143, 147, 151

Jaaniste, Joanna 8
Janus 4
Japanese Noh Theatre and Oshi
    Yoda 163
Jencks, Charles 7
Jennings, Sue 1, 10, 19, 77, 152, 157
Johnson, David Read 9–10, 149, 157
Jones, Phil 9, 39, 63, 76, 85, 149
Jung, C.G. 63

Kant, Immanuel 5
*Karuna* 123, 134
*Kha* 123, 127, 129–131, 133–135
Kim, Sung-Min 134; *Śunya: Immanent and Transcendent: Investigating Meanings of Void* 129–130
Klein, Melanie 98
Kranowitz, Carol Stock 36

Lahad, M. 166
Land, R. 87
Landy, Robert 19, 67, 85, 172
Laplanche, Jean 2–3
Lawrence, D.H. 151, 159
Lawson, B. 152
Lecoq, J. 60–63, 69
Levine, S.K. 17, 18, 20, 26
life force 126
liminality 23, 149–151, 153–154
Lively, Geneviève 24
*Lord Shiva* 129
Lucas, Catherine 126

Ma, Liwen 86–87
Madan, A. 37
*Magic Box* 157–159
Malchiodi, C. A. 77
malleable medium 50, 56
Mancia, M. 66
Mannoni, O. 51
Manzoni, Alessandro, *I promessi sposi* (*The Bethrothed*) 138
The Mask 64
Māui 35, 38
McNiff, Shaun 9–10
Meares, R. 93
mentalization 97
Merleau-Ponty, Maurice 5, 17–19
Messer, Sebastian 177–178
Meyer, J. 87
A Midsummer Night's Dream 150
Milner, Marion 50
Mitchell, Steve 93
Moore, R.L. 168, 173
'The Mother' from India 86
Mountford, A. 69–70
multimodality 115
Musicka-Williams, Amanda 10, 112

National Health Service 81
NDP *see* Neurodramatic play
Nemet-Pier, Lylian 47–48
Neolithic agricultural revolution 146

Neutral Mask 60–62, 66, 68–70
Neurodramatic play (NDP) 77
New Testament of the Bible 127
Nietzsche, F. 99
Nieuwenhuis, Marjin 1

Ogden, T. 2
Oliver, Mary 181
Olsen, Helge 45
Ovid 24; *Metamorphoses* 20

Pākehā 38–39, 40n9
Pendzik, Susana 9–10, 125, 153–154; *The theatre stage and the sacred space: a comparison* 9
Perec, George 4–5
Piaget, Jean 47
Pitruzzella, Salvo 9–10, 19–20, 22, 25–26; *spiritual magic* 151
place 2, 4–5, 10; pivotal 34; sacred 177; safe 46, 56, 98–99
Plato, *Timaeus* 5
play deprivation 38, 40
*Poiesis* 17–20, 22, 26–27
'power of Being' 127
preludial quality 1
Proshansky, Howard 42, 46
The Psychoanalytic Technique (Freud) 2
psychology/psychologist 4, 58, 180; analytical 63; behavioural 47; clinical 177; environmental 6–8, 42, 44, 46, 48, 55; social 47
psychotherapy 10, 166; group 64; nonverbal 1; traditional verbal 62

*The Question of Space* (2017) 1

Read, Gray 150, 156, 159
real life 45, 49, 51, 55, 83, 105, 112–115
recognition 106, 111–112, 115; aesthetic distance and 19; of commonalities 105; experiential 18
reflections 2, 4, 9–11, 25–27, 30, 42–43, 62, 80, 94–99, 104, 109, 134–135, 150, 155, 160, 176; aural 23; cognitive 115; evidence of 8; in-depth 178; spatial 177; spontaneous 63; substantial 131; visual 24
relational space 115; *see also* space
repetition 22–23, 92, 107–108
*Res cogitans* 145
*Res extensa* 145

Rizzolatti, Giacomo 144
Rogers, C. 94
Rogers, N. 165
Role-Play 64
Role Theory 64, 69
Romulus 146
Rousseau, Jean-Jacques 146
Roussillon, R. 50
*Rumpelstiltskin* 156
Ryle, Gilbert 145

safety 2, 35, 54–56, 64, 81, 91, 94–95,
    97–98, 100–101, 108, 166–167,
    169; emotional 151; psychological
    106–107, 151; space of 135
Saint Etienne Design Biennale 180
Scales, P. 153
scenography 43, 45, 55, 179–180
Schechner, Richard 8–10
Schiller, Friedrich 126
self-esteem 30, 46, 48, 57, 101
self-identity 46
Sendak, Maurice, 'Where the Wild
    Things are' 32–34
*Shunya* 123–124, 127–129, 131,
    133–135
*Shunya Purusha* 129
*Shunyata* 128–129
Singer, Michael A. 134
Slade, Peter 83–84; *Child Drama* 152
Smith, M. 75
Sobel, David 36
Sommer, Robert 44–45
space: active absence of 149–150;
    analytical 3; bridging 112–113;
    classroom 45, 113, 163, 170, 172;
    communal 177; concept of
    150–151; conditioned 163–165;
    containing 56, 60, 83; creative 56,
    154; drama therapeutic 45, 60, 65;
    dramatherapy 10, 18, 29, 34, 44,
    48, 50, 56–57, 69, 76, 79–80,
    83–85, 95, 104–107, 109–111,
    113, 117, 131, 151, 154, 165;
    dramatic 75–76, 80, 115–116,
    146–147, 167, 172; dream 62;
    educational 86, 177; embodied
    76–77; emotional 83; empty 123,
    128–129, 131, 147, 149, 164;
    enclosed 129–131; external 100,
    130, 133–134; good enough
    therapeutic 110; hammock and
    dream 51, 70; holding 99; hut

177; imaginal 104, 113–115;
    imaginary 166; imaginative 26,
    112; interpersonal 159;
    intersubjective 104–105, 149; is a
    doubt 4–6; legitimate 79; liminal
    53, 56, 79, 153, 159, 162–163,
    167–168, 172; liminoid 172; made
    of 144–146; magic 157; mask 177;
    mental health 78; narrative 107;
    neuropsychological 177; Neutral
    Mask 60–61; open 45;
    performance 80–81; performing
    114; peripersonal 144–145;
    personal 48, 65; personalization of
    47; physical 57, 81–83, 87, 104,
    106, 109–110, 112; play 9, 17–18,
    39, 45, 51, 91–94, 96–101, 105,
    108, 116–117, 157, 177, 180;
    poetic 23; potential 2, 17, 20, 38,
    101, 112, 116, 151; private 108;
    psychic 38, 54, 170;
    psychoanalytical 2–3; psychological
    104, 106–107; psycho-social 57;
    public 65; reflection 114; rehearsal
    105; relational 93, 97, 99, 104,
    106, 115, 159; and ritual
    151–153; ritual and spiritual 177;
    sacred 125, 131, 146–147, 154,
    162–165, 167–168, 170, 173; safe
    65, 80, 92, 98–99, 106–107, 162,
    165–166; safe enough 107, 169;
    scenographic and architectural
    177; self and other in 115; separate
    36; stage 3–4, 51, 53, 55, 149,
    162–163; temporary 162;
    theatrical 76; therapeutic 2, 9,
    35–36, 38–39, 45, 57, 82, 99,
    108, 110, 117, 123, 135, 165;
    therapy 3, 57, 125, 135, 162,
    165–166, 170–173; three-
    dimensional 42; transitional 56,
    99, 101, 112, 114, 151; utilitarian
    83; void 128–129
Spinoza, Baruch 145
spirit 129, 142–143; breath of 159
spirituality 126, 139, 142–143
spiritual realm 126–127
Sri Atmananda Krishna Menon 127
Stanislavski, C. 167
Sude, Michael E. 65
Svoboda, Robert 127
Swedenborg, Emanuel 126
Sweeney, Eliza 51, **52**, 96

Tagar, G.V., *The Skanda Purana* 128
Tāmaki Makaurau 34, 39, 40n7
tamariki 29, 31–37, 39, 40n5
tangata whenua 29, 40n1, 40n3
Taoist 123
Tayor, Judie 85
technology 135
territory 35; feelings of 56; notions of 47;
    sense of 47
Te Tai Tokerau 29, 34, 38, 40n4
Theory of Everything (TOE) 126
Tillich, Paul 127
Tipple, R. 166
trauma 38, 40, 47, 63, 68, 77, 91–92,
    95–96, 100, 107; abuse and 167;
    complex 152; intergenerational
    37–38
*Tribhuvan Threefold Psycho-spiritual
    Dramatherapy* 126
Tuan, Y.F. 76
Turner, Victor 78, 151, 153–154, 162,
    165, 172–173

UK Spiritual Crisis Network 126
*Ulu and the breadfruit tree* 156
United Kingdom (UK) 63, 81, 91, 155

Van Gennep, A. 151, 153–154, 162,
    164, 166, 172; *The Rites of
    Passage* 85
Vedanta 123, 127
*Vijnanabhairava* 128–129
*Vyoman* 123, 127–128

Wang Yang Ming 86
Warf, B. 10
whanau 40, 40n6
*whare* 34–35, 40n2
Whitehead, Derek, *Poiesis and Art-
    Making: A Way of Letting-Be* 130
Willshire, Amy 37
Winnicott, D.W. 17, 20, 38, 47, 54, 56,
    98, 101, 109–110, 151, 166
Witkin, Robert 20
Wolfsohn, Alfred 21
Wong, C. 45
Wood, A., *From the Upanishads* 127–128
Wordsworth, William 23–24
Wright, David Keir 21
*Wu* 129

Yalom, I. 166, 173